# Breast Cancer Answers
## Understanding and Fighting Breast Cancer

## Bruce A. Feinberg, D.O.

PRESIDENT/CHIEF EXECUTIVE OFFICER
GEORGIA CANCER SPECIALISTS

**LENZ BOOKS**

119 East Court Square, Suite 201
Decatur, Georgia 30030
www.lenzbooks.com

Lenz Books
119 East Court Sq.
Ste. 201
Decatur, GA 30030
www.lenzbooks.com

The authors, editor, and publisher have made every effort to provide accurate information. However, they are not responsible for errors, omissions, or for any outcomes related to the use of the contents of this book and take no responsibility for the use of the products described. Treatments and side effects described in this book may not be applicable to all patients; likewise, some patients may require a dose or experience a side effect that is not described herein. The reader should confer with his or her own physician regarding specific treatments and side effects. Drugs and medical devices are discussed that may have limited availability controlled by the Food and Drug Administration (FDA) for use only in a research study or clinical trial. The drug information presented has been derived from reference sources, recently published data, and pharmaceutical research data. Research, clinical practice, and government regulations often change the accepted standard in this field. When consideration is being given to use of any drug in the clinical setting, the healthcare provider or reader is responsible for determining FDA status of the drug, reading the package insert, reviewing prescribing information for the most up-to-date recommendations on dose, precautions, and contraindications, and determining the appropriate usage for the product. This is especially important in the case of drugs that are new or seldom used.

Breast Cancer Answers by Dr. Bruce Feinberg ISBN 978-0-9798560-1-3

**Production Credits**
Executive Editor: Richard J. Lenz
Associate Editor: Thomas Bell
Proofreader: Jamie Allen
Interior Illustrations: Bernie Kida, Jack Haley
Composition: Lenz, Decatur, Georgia
Original Cover Design: Scott Sanders
Printing and Binding: Asia Printing Co.
Cover Printing: Asia Printing Co.

Printed in Korea

10 9 8 7 6 5 4 3 2 1

*To Iris, Jon, Michael, Rachel, and Daniel,*
*Whose honesty keeps me humble;*
*Whose humor makes me laugh;*
*Whose love sustains me.*

# TABLE OF CONTENTS

# TABLE OF CONTENTS (continued)

# Preface

I am a medical oncologist, a doctor who specializes in the treatment of cancer. After more than 20 years of patient care, I remain amazed by how little most people know about how their bodies work. Despite access to information via books, television, and the Internet, most people know much more about how their cars and appliances work than they do about their bodies. Even more surprising are people's responses when their bodies are broken. Most people will not hesitate to get two opinions about a funny noise in their car engine before forking over $1,000 to fix it. Ironically, these same people will go to the first doctor to whom they are referred and undergo a $10,000 potentially life-threatening procedure with no questions asked.

The car is a mechanical machine, whereas the body is an organic machine, albeit more complex, but not impossible to understand. I have observed that my patients who understand how their bodies normally work and how they are affected by disease feel more in control when they face serious illness. No disease is more serious than cancer, and none makes a patient feel less in control. My hope is that this book provides patients, their families, and their caregivers with the information that they need to gain control and to participate in critical decision making. Hopefully, as an active participant in their care, patients can improve their outcomes.

*Dr. Bruce A. Feinberg*

# Acknowledgments

This book would not be possible without the guidance, support, knowledge, wisdom, and friendship of Richard Lenz. Richard, more than anyone, helped me translate the passion with which I educate my patients into a vehicle with which to educate breast cancer patients everywhere.

I am indebted to Melissa Faye Greene, whose validation of my work helped me persevere when I was at my lowest; Linda Loewenthal, who helped me understand the need to humanize science; and Estee Kunis, whose unqualified support gave me strength and confidence.

I thank Bernie Kida, who created the remarkable illustrations for Chapter 1 and helped set the narrative tone of the book. I would be remiss not to mention Chris Lybeer, a cancer survivor, friend, and constant resource who, among his many contributions, introduced me to Bernie. My appreciation is also extended to Jack Haley, who was able to capture Bernie's tone and complete the illustration content of the book.

To Cheryl Jones, Kristina Bowen, and Jan Galleshaw, my friends and colleagues: you are the epitome of a breast cancer physician. I would not have considered this book publishable without your review of the scientific content; thank you. To Chris Murphy, the best breast radiologist in Atlanta and a treasured community resource: my thanks for helping assemble the mammograms. To my physician colleagues at Georgia Cancer Specialists: your compassionate and knowledgeable patient care is a continuous source of pride that has helped me grow as both a physician and a human being.

To Scott Sanders who worked tirelessly to create the look, feel, and layout that make the narrative and illustrations flow effortlessly. To Deb Keen, my valued assistant, who never complains and who never lets me down. To John, Michael, and Ryan, and the rest of the foosball crew at Lenz Marketing: thank you for helping to create the comp that brought my vision to life.

Finally, I need to express my gratitude to the many patients who have entrusted their cancer care and their lives to my team of caregivers. I continue to be inspired by your courage and humbled by your grace. Physicians too often forget the gifts of knowledge and skill that allow them to help others during their time of need. I remember these gifts every day.

# How To Use This Book

Breast Cancer Answers is an outgrowth of my consultations with newly diagnosed breast cancer patients. Over the years it has become clear to me that simple illustrations were very effective in clarifying and reinforcing the explanations that I offered patients. My efforts to explain how the cancer began, how fast it was growing, whether it had spread, etc., were specifically enhanced with the illustrations. Despite the juvenile quality of my art, my patients often requested copies of the pencil drawings, as they helped them explain their situation to family and friends. One of my nurses suggested that I videotape a new patient discussion to improve my efficiency in the office, but I dismissed the notion as it seemed too impersonal. The suggestion did, however, trigger the thought that it would be wonderful if such a video or book were available for patients and families to have as a resource before and/or after the initial oncologic evaluation. I searched bookstores and web book retailers but could not find such a book. There seemed to be a real need for a breast cancer primer for patients. Breast Cancer Answers is designed to be such a primer. Each chapter builds on the information from the prior chapter. Illustrations accompany the narrative to reinforce and clarify the content. Keywords are in red, indicating that they can be found in the glossary for future reference.

My favorite book in medical school was an anatomy text that was illustrated with layered transparencies. With the pages in place, the image was of a human body. When the first transparency was lifted, the skin was peeled away, exposing the underlying musculature. When the second transparency was lifted, the muscles were gone, and the skeleton was exposed. Subsequent transparencies exposed the organs, the circulation, and the nervous systems. My hope is that this book peels away the confusion that confronts patients and their loved ones as each layer of the breast cancer problem is revealed.

# To the Newly Diagnosed Patient

You have just been informed you have cancer. You are in shock. Your life is suddenly turned upside down. Don't panic! As ridiculous as it sounds, this is the best advice I can offer. To overcome the panic, you have to understand what is happening and what is going to happen to you. Your panic is rooted in the fear of the unknown and an irrational response to a situation of which you have no knowledge, no experience, and no control. Worse, you have only limited knowledge or indirect experience from cancer situations that are totally unrelated to the one that you are experiencing now. You are a newly diagnosed breast cancer patient, and your father's lung cancer and Aunt Ethel's leukemia are as different in behavior and outcome as are ice cream and artichokes.

In order not to panic and to gain control, you need to be educated about what has happened to your body and what should be anticipated. Unfortunately, seeking knowledge from well-intentioned friends and family or via the Internet is more likely to confuse than to comfort. Do not panic! With this book, the knowledge that you need to approach this disease with a positive attitude is provided.

Many types of cancer exist. With all cancers, cells in the body change and grow out of control. Usually, the multiplying cancer cells form a lump called a cancerous tumor. Cancerous tumors are also called malignant tumors. Sometimes malignant tumor cells can break away from the mass and travel through the bloodstream or lymphatic system to other parts of the body. This process is called metastasis. Not all tumors are cancerous. Those that are not are called benign. Cells from benign tumors do not spread to other parts of the body.

These statements seem straightforward enough and are probably adequate for the majority of people who have not encountered the most dreaded three words in the human language: You have cancer! However, when I am in the unfortunate situation of having to say these words to a new patient and his or her anxious loved ones, this explanation is woefully inadequate. Those involved need to know so much more. The questions are endless: Where did it come from? Why did it happen to me? When did it start? How far has it gone? How big is it? Has it spread? How can it be stopped, treated, and cured? For those who are actively battling breast cancer or who are supporting a spouse, child, parent, loved one, or friend who is suffering with breast cancer, this book is for you. This is the what, where, when, why, and how of breast cancer that hopefully will make sense of everything that you have heard, seen, been through, or are about to experience. In short, I hope to answer all of the questions about breast cancer that you may have—hence the title, Breast Cancer Answers.

Cancer is the most complex of human diseases. It begins with a step-by-step transformation of a single human cell. Because there are over 200 types of cells in the human body, over 200 types of cancer exist, each one distinct. How can we begin to understand the more than 200 most complex human diseases? First, we turn our attention to just one cancer, breast cancer. Then, we begin as the cancer does, with a single cell. We begin by examining the origin of a human cell and the progression to the 200 different types of cells that make up a complete body. We learn about the cells that make up the breast and their normal structure and function. We examine how their behavior changes as they transform into a cancerous or malignant state. We discuss what causes this transformation as we explore cellular DNA, the genetic blueprint, or operating code that governs the cell's behavior. We describe the natural history of breast cancer and how we use this knowledge to predict a cancer's course and plan its therapy. We present the current strategies that medical science uses to both treat and prevent cancer. Finally, we try to make sense of the gobbledy gook of jargon, terms, and statistics that can either paralyze patients with fear or confuse them with false expectations.

Read this book cover to cover. Do not skip. Do not browse. Do not wander. I have specifically written this book to provide a step-by-step understanding of breast cancer. Like the layered transparencies of my college anatomy text that peeled away the external structure to reveal the inner workings, this book explains the transformation from the normal breast to breast cancer with all of its implications. The narrative is accompanied by illustrations that will assist you as you journey through the complicated world of medical jargon and statistics. Important key words and terms are in red and can be found in the glossary. Take pauses to digest each chapter; read, go back, and reread if needed, but read methodically chapter by chapter. Use the illustrations found in each chapter to clarify and reinforce the narrative. This book is designed to be read in one evening and is going to eliminate hours, days, and weeks of emotional agony. Don't panic! Read this book!

# SECTION 1

# Before the Surgery

# Introduction

Medical oncologists are physicians who take care of cancer patients. The most common cancers are those that originate in the body's organs, such as the colon, prostate, lung, and breast. Rarely does a week go by that I do not see a new patient with a recently diagnosed breast cancer.

Jill was 37 years old. She was the mother of Josh and Amy, ages 7 and 9 years, and wife to Greg for 10 years. Life had been good. Jill worked as a lawyer until Josh was born and had recently returned to work part-time for a community agency. Eight weeks prior, Jill had had her annual routine physical and pap smear with her gynecologist, Dr. Scott. Almost as an afterthought, Dr. Scott suggested that she might consider getting a baseline mammogram. He does not normally recommend a baseline mammogram until his patients are 40 years old, which is considered the standard of care unless the patient has had an abnormal exam or a family history of breast cancer; Jill had neither. Maybe a remote patient experience or an article that he had recently read in one of his medical journals triggered the suggestion. He assured Jill that he was not hiding anything from her; her breast exam was very unremarkable. "We'll get a baseline now and then at age 40 begin annual surveillance," he said. It all seemed so innocent and matter of fact.

Jill scheduled the mammogram to be done in five weeks when there was a convenient opening at the Women's Health Imaging Center. Jill had little trepidation; it was, after all, routine, like her annual pap smear. The mammogram was a bit uncomfortable, and although the procedure took only a few minutes, getting to and from the imaging center, checking in, and waiting to be examined consumed half of the day. By the time Josh and Amy got home from school, the experience was forgotten. She was told that a nurse from Dr. Scott's office would call in a few weeks to tell her that the mammogram was okay, as the office nurse does after her annual pap smear.

Dr. Scott himself called the next day. Jill's apprehension began with the sound of his voice, and panic erupted as he explained that there was an abnormality on the mammogram. He wanted her to go back to the imaging center that afternoon for some additional mammograms and an ultrasound. She put down the phone, called Greg, and started to cry. They met at the imaging center. After the tests, the radiologist began to explain the findings. The radiologist showed Jill and Greg the mammogram abnormalities on a computer screen. Jill spoke to Dr. Scott, and an appointment was made to see a breast surgeon three days later. All of her fears were supposed to be assuaged by Dr. Scott's reassurances: "It's probably nothing, but we want to be sure," and "God forbid, if it is anything, you are very lucky because it was found early." It! "The 'it' the doctors are speaking of is cancer." Jill thought, "What kind of luck is that? I am 37, with two small children and I have cancer."

In shock and silence, Jill and Greg drove home. The kids returned home from school, and Jill and Greg compartmentalized their anguish. That evening, after Josh and Amy went to sleep, Jill began making phone calls to the few friends and family who she knew had some personal experience with cancer. Doctors, hospitals, Internet sites, and alternative therapies were recommended with conviction. Jill was overwhelmed. She took a deep breath and tried to sort out what was happening. She resolved to proceed with Dr. Scott's plan but also to seek a second opinion. In the morning, she made an appointment with a second surgeon.

By the time I met Jill and Greg, three weeks had elapsed since that infamous day when the possibility of having cancer was introduced into their good life. A biopsy had been performed on the right breast. Two surgical opinions rendered, and a reconstructive surgery evaluation scheduled. Despite the time, energy, and multiple professional opinions, Jill and Greg, an intelligent, well-educated couple, had more questions than answers. They were in my office because the second surgeon raised the possibility that Jill might be genetically predisposed to breast cancer. Before making a final decision regarding the type of breast surgery, the second surgeon suggested that genetic testing should be performed. Jill and Greg thought they were referred to me to discuss genetic testing in more detail. They were completely surprised when I mentioned that chemotherapy might be needed after surgery.

The questions and concerns were endless. Which surgical option was best? Lumpectomy, mastectomy, or bilateral mastectomy? Should the reconstruction be immediate or delayed, and what kind of reconstruction would be best? Would radiation therapy be necessary, and if so, would it impact the choice and timing of reconstruction? Why would she need chemotherapy after surgery? Why had the other doctors not mentioned it, and if it was needed, what kind and for how long? Was there a genetic predisposition of cancer? Why did it happen? When did it happen? How did it happen? Would it impact her children?

I have been seeing couples like Jill and Greg every week for nearly 20 years. I share their anguish; I see their pain. They had suffered through three weeks of anxiety and fear—an emotional suffering that was to continue for possibly another two to three weeks until the results of surgery would dictate final treatment recommendations. Despite family and friends, the physician consultations, books, and the Internet, patients like Jill and Greg remain in the isolation of the unknown, their minds inextricably fixating on the worst-case scenario. Jill and Greg and the tens of thousands of people like them cannot find comfort, or calm their irrational fear until they understand the biological process related to this odyssey. They need the time to digest the myriad of pieces of information thrown at them, and they need the facts filtered from the fiction. They need the information accessible to digest at their pace, not in the 30 minutes allotted to them in the doctor's office. That is what this book does. This book is for Jill and Greg, their parents and siblings, their caring friends, and their children. It is for the 250,000 newly diagnosed breast cancer patients in the United States this year and for the more than three million women living after a diagnosis of breast cancer.

Let me begin by explaining to you, as I explained to Jill and Greg, what happened to her body and how it led to a breast cancer diagnosis.

# Chapter One

# The Basic Science of Breast Cancer

## The Cell

I have always believed that to understand what really happens to the body when it is stricken with disease you have to have some basic understanding of biology as well as human anatomy and physiology. Unfortunately, discussing such subjects can be rather dry and complicated. During such discussions my patients often echo my wife, who is fond of saying, "Just tell me the time, not how to build a clock." Even as I considered writing the **Cancer Answers** series, I was still struggling to find metaphors and imagery that would help my patients and possible readers grasp the biologic principles that are critical to understanding how cancers begin and grow. Divine providence seemed to intervene when my then 7-year-old son, Daniel, asked if I would speak to his second-grade class. He explained that the class was completing a study unit entitled "Jobs," and parents were encouraged to visit the class and talk about their work. After a pregnant pause, I told him I was delighted to speak, but I was not quite sure whether talking about cancer was appropriate for 7-year-olds. Daniel assuaged my concerns, telling me that other parents who were physicians had already presented. One child's mother explained how she kept sick people asleep while they had surgery, and another child's father talked about how he helped people to breathe better. The gauntlet was thrown: if an anesthesiologist and a pulmonologist could do it, then so could a medical oncologist. I contacted Daniel's teacher and arranged my visit. The day approached, and I was beginning to panic that there was just no way to explain cancer to 7-year-old children. To have any hope of understanding cancer and its treatment, you have to understand that animals are made from cells, that cells can transform and grow out of control, and that medicines are

Figure 1-1 The Lego—the Perfect Metaphor for the Cell

available that can kill these transformed, bad-behaving cells without harming the good cells that keep us alive. Unfortunately, these kids were in second grade and did not even know what a cell was.

I went to Daniel's bedroom to confess my dilemma. Daniel was on the floor with his Legos splayed about him. When I saw the hundreds of Legos in every color, shape, and size joined in various ways to create cars, houses, and planes, I had an epiphany. The Lego was the perfect metaphor for a cell (Figure 1-1).

Figure 1-2: Assorted Legos

In Legoland, the Lego is the basic building block. Hundreds of different types of Legos, when appropriately combined, can create an infinite variety of structures. You can take Legos of just one variety and stack them side by side and up and down to create a wall. Add two windows and a door, and create the completed front wall of a house. After a child builds three sidewalls and secures them with a floor and a roof, the house takes on a recognizable appearance. Eureka, my problem was solved (Figure 1-2).

I explained to Daniel that while the Lego is the basic building block of Legoland, the cell is the basic building block of organic life (living creatures). The cell is called the origin of life because one cell gives rise to the billions of cells that make the complete animal. Like Legos, the billions of cells are not identical in appearance but rather fall into a few hundred different types: hair cells, skin cells, blood cells, etc. (Figure 1-3).

Figure 1-3: Assorted Cells

The formation of a human body, like any mammal's body, begins with the meeting of a sperm and an egg. The sperm fertil-

Figure 1-4:
The Origin of Life

Figure 1-5:
Cellular Division

izes the egg, creating the first cell, the beginning of a human body (Figure 1-4). This cell then divides to make two cells. Two cells divide to make four, and then those cells continue to divide until there is a cluster of cells (Figure 1-5). Initially, all of the cells in the cluster are identical. Next, these identical cells begin a process in which they become the more than 200 different types of cells that make the human body complete. This process is called DIFFERENTIATION; the cells differentiate or become different types. This early developing human is called an EMBRYO.

The process of differentiation in the developing embryo begins with these clustered cells organizing into three layers: an outer layer called the ECTODERM, an inner layer called the ENDODERM, and a middle layer called the MESODERM. These three layers of cells are in turn encased in a layer of cells that will give rise to the placenta. The outer of these three layers, the ectoderm, differentiates into skin and nerve cells. The middle layer, the mesoderm, differentiates into blood, muscle, and bone cells. The inner layer, the endoderm, differentiates into the cells that comprise all of the body's organs (Figure 1-6).

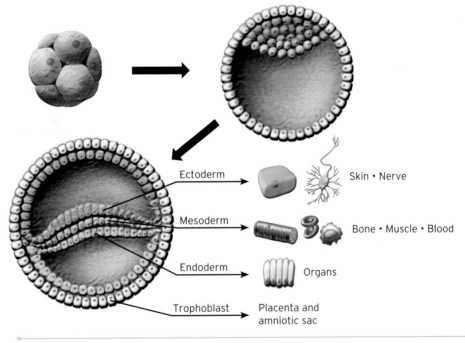

Figure 1-6: Cellular Differentiation

Imagine Legoland being alive. In the beginning, there was one small, rectangular, white Lego. Then there were a bunch of small, rectangular, white Legos; then white Legos morphed into three groups—white, red, and blue rectangles.

Primitively speaking, all of your body's organ cells begin with the endoderm layer: they have a common origin and are structurally similar. This is a very important point, as we will later see. As these primitive cells further differentiate and mature, their structure and function assume that of adult cells. Mature cells progress from individual cells to sheets of cells. The sheets of cells then organize to form TISSUES. Different types of tissues combine to form organs. Organs connect to create systems, (e.g., the reproductive system, gastrointestinal system.) Finally, the systems are arranged within a musculoskeletal framework supported by a circulatory and nervous system.

Returning to our Legoland metaphor, the white, red, and blue Legos have now morphed into hundreds of different types. There are billions of each type, trillions of Legos in all. Some Legos have been assembled into a wall (like sheets of cells forming tissues). Doors and windows have been added to the wall to make the front of a house (like an organ), and roofs, floors, walls, and more have been organized to make a complete house (like a complete human being).

Daniel was an attentive and courteous listener as I expounded gleefully, progressing from Legos and cells to cancer and treatment. When I finished my diatribe, gratified to have found the long-sought metaphor, I asked Daniel what he thought. He said that he liked the Lego part but that I definitely needed to bring some kind of neat machine, like the breathing thing with the balls that go up and down that the lung doctor demonstrated. Also, I needed to bring a giveaway such as gloves or masks or maybe pencils with my name on it. I left Daniel's room defeated, feeling small and humbled. I went to my office with hopes of finding something appropriate to give 15 second graders, pondering what kind of cancer machine I could demonstrate.

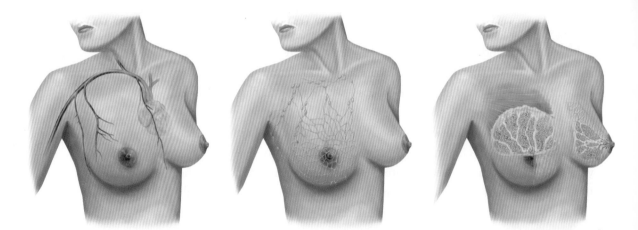

Figure 1-7 A:
Breast: Blood Supply

Figure 1-7 B:
Breast: Lymphatic Drainage

Figure 1-7 C:
Breast: Connective Tissue and Fat

# The Breast: Normal Structure and Function

J ill and Greg were among the first patients to see my Legos demonstration, and it was a success. Not only did they not think I was crazy, but it helped them to understand cells. The next step was to explain why humans have breasts and what kinds of cells comprise them.

Unlike the Legos that I have been using for illustration, cells not only have structure, they also have function and are alive. To stay alive, cells must eat and breathe; blood provides the oxygen and food. Like the cells that comprise them, animals have to eat and breathe; they also have to reproduce or their species will become extinct. The newborns that result from reproduction must be fed before they can feed themselves. Humans are equipped with specialized cells organized into an organ that can nourish the newborn. That organ is the breast.

Recall from the last chapter that cells organize into tissues and tissues combine to make organs. All organs, including the breast, require VASCULAR TISSUE to carry blood with its nutrients, oxygen and glucose. All organs have LYMPHATIC TISSUE to transport lymph fluid and immune cells, irrigating and cleansing all the cells of the organ, removing the bacteria and viruses so they can be trapped and destroyed within nearby filters called LYMPH NODES. All organs must be held in place by some sort of CONNECTIVE TISSUE (e.g., muscle, tendon, ligament). And all organs are surrounded by a FATTY TISSUE.

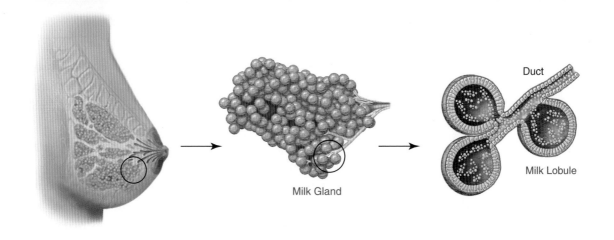

Figure 1-8: Mammary Tissue Magnified

(Figure 1.7) What makes each organ unique is the specialized tissue endowing its unique function.

The breast is not an appendage like a hand or an arm. It is an organ, like a lung, liver, or kidney. You can think of an organ as having a bodily function, like the lung taking in oxygen or the kidney removing waste. The function of the breast is to produce milk for the newborn. Milk production, or LACTATION, requires two cellular structures: the LOBULES, which make the milk, and the DUCTS, a system of tubes that carry the milk to the nipple. The lobule cells produce the milk, which then drips into the tubes created by the duct cells so that it can flow to the nipple.

The specialized, functional tissue in the breast that contains the lobules and the ducts is called MAMMARY TISSUE; a MAMMOGRAM is simply an x-ray of mammary tissue. Mammary tissue—with its blood supply and lymphatic drainage, the fibrous or connective tissue that holds it all together, the fat cells that fill the gaps, and the overlying skin—is what makes the organ called a breast. The diseases referred to as breast cancer develop in the mammary tissue within the breast. All human beings have breasts with mammary tissue, but men's breasts remain undeveloped in the absence of ESTROGENS at puberty.

Under low-power magnification, the mammary tissue is organized like bunches of grapes. Metaphorically, the grapes are the lobules, clustered in bunches, dripping milk into their hollow stems, which are the ducts. A mammary duct under higher power magnification appears as a tubelike structure, a living tube. The wall of the tube is made of cells. All of the bunches and all of the stems are connected to a common vine, the nipple. (Figure 1-8)

Throughout a woman's adult life, beginning with the start of her menstrual years, the mammary tissue is under constant stress. Month after month, the changes in a woman's HORMONE levels cause changes in the breast. These changes are physical, as well as hormonal. Before the menstrual period, the breasts become tender and swollen as the ducts dilate and the lobules enlarge in preparation for milk production if a pregnancy should occur.

Except for the interruptions of pregnancy and postpartum lactation stimulated by breastfeeding, these cyclical physical and hormonal stresses will occur for 30 to 40 years. The declining estrogen production of midlife (PERI-MENOPAUSE) causes a regression or shrinkage of mammary tissue and an increase in the fat content of the breast. The cyclical physical and hormonal changes cease at MENOPAUSE despite the fact that a woman's body continues to produce low levels of estrogen. (Yes, postmenopausal women still make estrogen, as is discussed later.)

Jill began menstruating at the age of 13 years, nearly 25 years ago. She had never thought about her breasts as milk-making machines working continuously, albeit mostly in standby mode, for over a quarter century. Could decades of physical and hormonal stress have caused serious problems in her mammary tissue?

## Carcinogenesis

Throughout your lifetime cells are continuously injured and repaired. Bruises, scrapes, cuts, burns, infections, chapped lips, and tongues burned by pizza cheese and hot coffee are examples of the myriad everyday cellular injuries that you experience. Your body has the remarkable ability to repair this cellular damage and does so in a constant, ongoing process. Some cellular damage is below the surface, caused by the tobacco smoke that we inhale, the chemicals in the food that we eat, the radiation from the sun, and the natural internal, physical, chemical, and hormonal stresses that are part and parcel of being alive. Sometimes, if the injuries are chronic or recurrent, or if there is a genetic predisposing defect, the body is unable to repair the cellular injury. The body's failure or inability to repair cellular injury can lead to cancer. The process by which the failed repair of cellular injury leads to cancer is called CARCINOGENESIS.

In the beginning of this chapter, I mentioned that all of the body's specialized organ tissue has a common origin in the cells of the endoderm of the developing embryo. As these primitive cells mature, they retain certain common features, giving organ tissue a similar appearance under the microscope. The microscopic appearance is often referred to as GLANDULAR, which means something different than what you might think. To a PATHOLOGIST, glandular tissue refers to a group of cells that are organized so that they can either take in nutrients (absorb) or release chemicals needed to maintain normal body function (secrete). The cell type common to these glandular tissues is called an EPITHELIAL CELL. Epithelial cells are flat where they connect organs to the outside, such as at the mouth and anus. And they are cube-shaped in the organs that are secretory, such as the breast, prostate, and pancreas: and they are an elongated cube or column-shaped in the organs that absorb nutrients, such as the colon and small intestine. When flat epithelial cells transform into cancer, they are called SQUAMOUS CELL CARCINOMA. When cuboidal or columnar epithelial cells transform into cancer, they are called ADENOCARCINOMA.

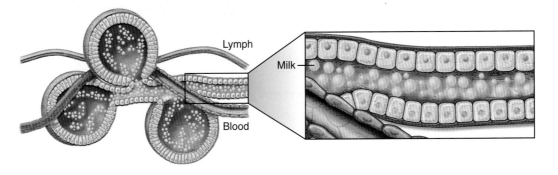

Figure 1-9: Normal Duct Cells

The glandular tissue of the breast, comprised of lobules and ducts, is called mammary tissue; it makes or secretes milk for the newborn baby (Figure 1-9). Researchers have begun to unravel the mystery of the genetic, molecular, and cellular changes that lead to the carcinogenesis of mammary tissue. As I explain in Chapter 2, these injuries are not superficial and are not on the surface of the cell. Rather, these changes occur deep within the guts of the cell, in its nucleus and DNA, changing the cell's appearance, behavior, and very essence. They can literally turn a cell from its well-behaved and orderly Dr. Jekyll into Mr. Hyde, wreaking havoc and chaos. The process of transformation from Jekyll to Hyde is predictable, often slow, but always relentless.

When mammary cells transform into cancer, it is referred to as ADENO-CARCINOMA OF THE BREAST. The process begins with the hormonal and physical stress on the duct cells, as the ducts dilate and then contract with each normal menstrual cycle. These stresses lead to irritation and then injury of the duct cells. If the body is unable to repair the injured cells, new cells are added to the injured ones, resulting in an overgrowth of duct cells, which is called DUCTAL HYPERPLASIA (Figure 1.10).

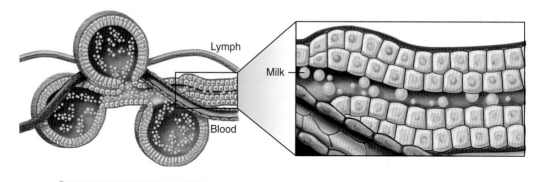

Figure 1-10: Ductal Hyperplasia

As the cells continue to overgrow, they become unstable, altering their appearance and behavior. The cells become larger and less uniform, their growth pattern less organized. At this point, pathologists call the overgrowth ATYPICAL DUCTAL HYPERPLASIA (Figure 1.11).

Continued stress, cellular injury, and repair process mistakes result in what are called MUTATIONS (physical changes in cellular DNA, as described

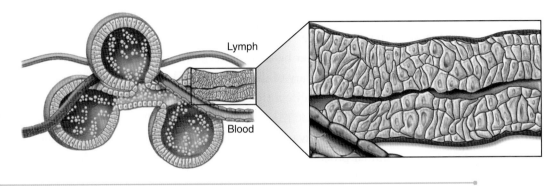

Figure 1-11: Atypical Hyperplasia

in more detail later in this chapter), which lead to the creation of more aggressive cells. These more aggressive cells may so overgrow that they fill the entire duct space, may extend down the duct space into the lobule space, then may begin to distort and swell the duct. The abnormal cell growth and behavior may also result in small deposits of calcium referred to as MICRO-CALCIFICATIONS. The packed and swollen ducts with their microcalcification may become large enough that they can be felt on examination or seen on a mammogram. These are the characteristics of the earliest form of cancer, what is technically called DUCTAL CARCINOMA IN SITU (duct cancer within place) or DCIS (Figure 1.12). Other terms used to describe this condition are INTRADUCTAL CANCER and NONINVASIVE DUCTAL CANCER.

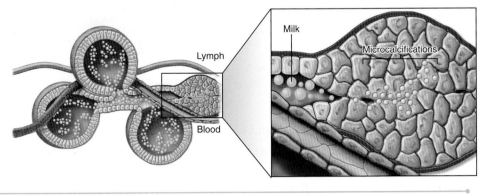

Figure 1-12: Ductal Carcinoma in Situ

Unfortunately, patients and doctors do not always observe distortion, lumps, or other changes on an exam or microcalcification on a mammogram. Not all women get mammograms, see their physician for an annual exam, or perform self-exams. Finally, neither the physical exam nor mammography is foolproof. If DCIS remains undetected, the next event that can occur is an even more aggressive change. These unstable, mutated duct cells that have met the first criteria of cancer by their pattern of intraductal overgrowth no longer respect the boundary of the duct wall. They invade or infiltrate through the duct wall (visualize a tree root growing through the street or sidewalk). This INVASIVE DUCTAL CARCINOMA, or INFILTRATING DUCTAL CARCINOMA, is the most advanced form of cancer within the breast (Figure 1.13). (A very similar process may occur within the lobule cells leading to both LOBULAR CARCINOMA IN SITU and INVASIVE LOBULAR CANCER. However, pure lobular cancer is far less common, and the progression of lobular carcinoma in situ to invasive cancer is less clear. So we will focus on DCIS and invasive ductal cancer.)

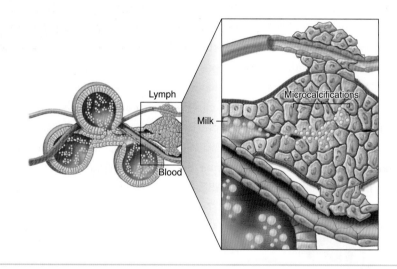

Figure 1-13: Early Invasion Ductal Carcinoma

The more I explained to Jill and Greg, the more questions they had. If hormonal and physical stress occurs in the breasts of all women, then why do all women not develop breast cancer? If these same stresses occur throughout both breasts and involve all mammary ducts, then why do only some ducts transform? I advised a deep breath and patience because I was just about to explain how physical and hormonal stress cause cellular transformation and initiate the cascade of events that result in cancer. In order to understand the how and why of carcinogenesis, one needs to understand the inner workings of a cell—its GENETIC CODE.

# Genetics

All human cells have a similar design: an outer membrane covering a gelatinous liquid, cytoplasm, within which is a central core structure, the NUCLEUS. The image is that of a Tootsie Pop where the wrapper is the cell membrane, the lollypop candy is the cytoplasm, and the Tootsie Roll is the nucleus (Figure 1-14). Within the nucleus resides the blueprint or operating code of not only the cell but also of the entire organism.

Figure 1-14: The Cell as a Tootsie Pop

Like computer software written in special binary code, the operating code of living organisms is written in a special language called DNA, which is actually a chemical code comprised of four characters called NUCLEOSIDE BASES. DNA is a unique code language that, once translated, instructs the cell to build PROTEINS. Proteins are the cell's machines that bring food into the cell, remove waste from the cell, repair the cell after injury, prepare the cell for growth and division, etc.

Like many other types of machines that we are more familiar with, proteins may have many different functions but are all structurally related. Automobiles, tractors, speedboats, and helicopters are very different forms of transportation but are all propelled by an internal combustion engine. Refrigerators, blenders, washers, and coffee grinders are very different appliances, but they are all powered by an electric motor. Computers, cell phones, digital cameras, and CD players perform different functions, but they are all controlled by a microprocessor chip. Like each of these examples of inorganic machines, proteins are the workhorses of organic machines and the cells that comprise them. The blueprint for each protein is encrypted in the DNA code.

By definition, a code must be broken or translated for the encrypted message to be understood. The DNA message for protein building requires not only translation, but also transportation from the nucleus to the cytoplasm where the proteins are manufactured. The translation and subsequent transport of the encrypted DNA message is facilitated by another nucleoside base language called RNA. The DNA message is translated to RNA, which leaves the nucleus and travels to the cytoplasm where it docks with a structure called a RIBOSOME, the protein-manufacturing factory.

The chemical building blocks of proteins are called AMINO ACIDS. Amino acids are chemically linked one to another according to the instructions of the DNA message. Let me try to summarize in a single statement: *Amino acids in the cytoplasm are assembled into proteins by the ribosome under the direction of an RNA message, which is the translation of a DNA code sequence from within the nucleus* (Figure 1-15).

Figure 1-15: The Biochemical Basis of Life: DNA-RNA-Protein. Amino acids in the cytoplasm are assembled into proteins by the ribosome under the direction of an RNA message, which is the translation of a DNA code sequence from within the nucleus. Every cell in the body has the complete manual of information (genome) stored in its library (nucleus).

A complete DNA sequence that encodes a protein is called a GENE. Genes are clustered into long strands of DNA called CHROMOSOMES, which are made even longer because these genes are also separated from one another by non-message base sequences. There are 46 chromosomes in a normal human cell, 23 contributed by the father via the sperm and 23 contributed by the mother via the egg. The chromosomes are arranged in 23 pairs. Scientists now believe that there are between 20,000 and 40,000 genes necessary for human life, making it likely that there are approximately 1,000 to 2,000 genes per chromosome pair.

Think of this genetic operating system, or GENOME, as the body's complete information encyclopedia or, better still, the body's owner's manual. Everything needed to build, operate, and repair the body is written in the manual, with a copy residing in each cell. The encyclopedic owner's manual ... is comprised of 23 volumes (chromosome pairs), each 1,000–2,000 chapters long (genes) composed in a four-character code language (DNA) requiring billions of characters (nucleoside bases) in all. *Every cell in the body has the complete manual of information (genome) stored in its library (nucleus),* but only certain volumes are off the shelf at any one time, opened to specific chapters as the genetic needs dictate. Genes for hair color are not turned on in blood cells, and genes to produce HEMOGLOBIN are not turned on in hair cells. Beginning in the embryo and throughout cellular differentiation, fetal maturation, growth, and development, messages are turned on and off in a complex system of signals and responses. For the messages and signaling to work properly, every cell needs to have its billions of characters (nucleoside bases) in the correct sequence, ready for the moment when one of the volumes is taken off the shelf and opened to a chapter to be translated.

A mistake in a base sequence is called a MUTATION. Mutations can occur in a variety of ways. Let's use that encyclopedic owner's manual metaphor to illustrate the point. Sometimes information passed on from a parent is incorrect, causing some of the chapters to have wrong information. Such genetic mutations are called HEREDITARY MUTATIONS. Sometimes there is a misprint at the factory (embryo or fetus), leading to incorrect information in some of the chapters. Such genetic mutations are called CONGENITAL MUTATIONS. Most commonly, the original information and printing are correct, but from years of use and handling, print becomes smudged, paper stained, or pages torn, leading to incorrect messages. Such genetic mutations are called ACQUIRED MUTATIONS.

Genetic defects or mutations that cause a cell to reproduce uncontrollably and invade surrounding structures are what cause cancer. Many forms of cellular injury like those caused by chemicals and radiation lead to the types of mutations that cause carcinogenesis. Acquired mutations rarely occur from a single insult but rather from repeated insult and injury such as decades of sun exposure, years of tobacco use, chronic irritation from fecal waste, decades of cyclic hormonal stress, or just living. Thus, all cancers are consequences of genetic mutations, but few, approximately 10%, are hereditary. Most cancers are the result of acquired genetic mutations (Figure 1-16).

Figure 1-16: Relationship of Mutational Events to Carcinogenesis

Was Jill's breast cancer hereditary? Neither Jill's mother nor her sister had a history of breast cancer. She was of Ashkenazi Jewish ancestry, which she knew was a RISK FACTOR. She also knew her age at diagnosis, less than 40 years, suggested that her risk of hereditary breast cancer was greater than 10%. This is an important piece of information as it indicates a higher probability of future breast cancers and could influence choice of surgery for someone like Jill. If you are likely to develop another cancer in the same or opposite breast, you may choose not to keep your breasts but rather have them both removed (more discussion in Chapter 3).

Breast cancer, like the majority of adult cancers, most often occurs in the sixth and seventh decades of life and is predominantly the result of acquired mutations brought about by years of cellular stress and injury. The transformation to cancer is slow, taking years or decades as gene after gene is mutated until one day the mutations are extensive enough to meet the criteria that define cancer. The most serious mutations are those that lead to cells invading surrounding structures and spreading through the blood and lymph circulations, as is described next.

## Invasion and Metastases

Jill's normal breast exam, an absence of symptoms, and minimal mammographic abnormalities suggested that her cancer was found early, before it was invasive, at the stage of progression called DCIS. Unfortunately, the biopsy revealed a small area of invasive cancer cells (Figure 1-17). What makes invasive breast cancer more problematic is the possibility of cancer cells entering into the blood. As I explained earlier, the duct is a living tissue composed of cells. Every cell must have a blood supply to survive. Therefore,

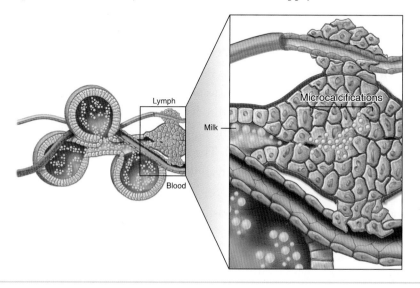

Figure 1-17: Early Invasive Ductal Carcinoma

supporting the mammary tissue are a matrix of blood vessels sending off small branches that nourish each of the living cells that make up the duct and the lobule. As the invasive cancer grows through or infiltrates the wall of the duct, it may also grow through or infiltrate the wall of a nearby blood vessel. Once exposed to the blood stream, cancer cells may break free from the growing cluster (TUMOR), gaining access to the blood circulation as it flows through the breast (Figure 1.18).

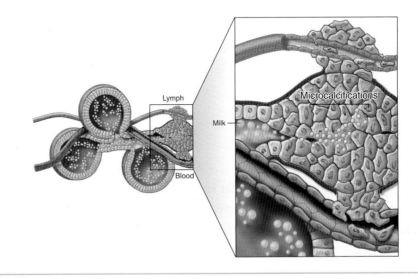

Figure 1-18: Vascular and Lymphatic Invasion

If cancer cells or cell clusters survive in the blood circulation, they may adhere or anchor to the wall of a blood vessel anywhere in the body and there begin a new nest of growing cancer cells (Figure 1.19). This nest may then invade through the blood vessel wall (just as it originally invaded through the duct wall). This nest may then extend through the vessel wall into the organ in which that blood vessel is located (the lung, the liver, etc.), forming a cancerous tumor in that organ (Figure 1.20). The nest of breast cancer cells—anchored into a blood vessel of another organ where it then forms a cancerous tumor—is what doctors call a METASTASIS. (A similar process can occur within the lymph circulation of the breast, as explained in Chapter 3.)

The overriding concern for patients with infiltrating or invasive breast cancer, and the doctors who treat them, is whether breast cancer cells have escaped into the circulation and might develop into METASTASES. The mission of the cancer doctor is to determine the risk of metastases in order to either do something preemptively to destroy the escaping cells before they anchor, nest, and/or invade another organ (ADJUVANT THERAPY) or to treat the metastases if they can be identified or are readily apparent (METASTATIC THERAPY).

Fortunately for Jill, like most women whose cancer is diagnosed by screening mammogram, even when the cancer is invasive, cure is more likely if it is found early.

Let us return to Jill's exam, mammogram, and biopsy to understand better what occurred before she was referred. We'll also answer those nagging questions about why doctors cannot always find breast cancer during their exam, at what age women should begin screening mammograms, and why biopsies are needed before surgery.

Figure 1-19: Anchored Tumor Cells

Figure 1-20: Metastases

# Chapter Two

# Diagnosing Breast Cancer

The ultimate goal of cancer research is to prevent the disease the way vaccination has eradicated polio and smallpox. In the absence of a definitive prevention strategy, medical science's best efforts have been applied to finding or SCREENING for the disease early enough so that it is curable in virtually 100% of those in whom it is found. Unfortunately, some cancer screening tests that attempt to find the cancer early, before it produces symptoms and when it is curable, have had mixed success. Unlike the unquestioned success of the pap smear in allowing the early detection and cure of cervix cancer, colonoscopy in permitting the early detection and cure of colon cancer, and PSA (prostate specific antigen) testing in permitting the early detection and cure of prostate cancer, the screenings for breast, lung, and other cancers remain controversial.

It seems not a month goes by without a major news story about a scientific study calling into question the value of breast exams and mammograms. The elaborate and often complex scientific studies are reduced to 30-second sound bites that give the impression that women might as well just roll the dice when it comes to early detection of breast cancer. Although I appreciate the science and recognize the need to scrutinize both the cost and value of all medical interventions, I remain steadfast in my support of early detection by the best proven means available, which today are manual breast examination and mammography.

My logic is simple: Cancer evolves from a precancerous state to a noninvasive state to an invasive state. The greater the number of cancer cells, the greater the risk of mutation to an invasive state. The greater the number of invasive cells, the greater the risk of those invading cells escaping into the circulation. The greater the number of cells in the circulation, the greater

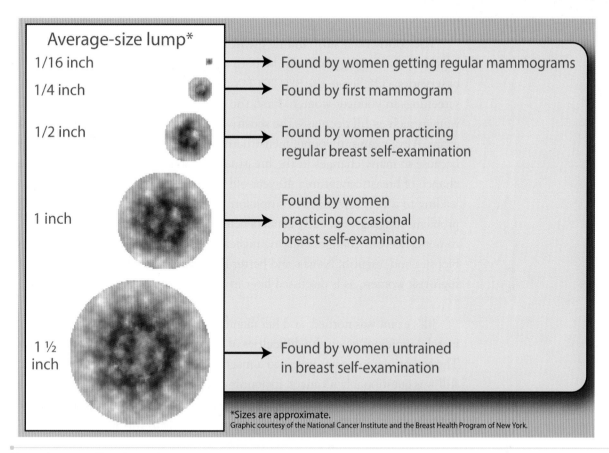

Average-size lump*

1/16 inch → Found by women getting regular mammograms

1/4 inch → Found by first mammogram

1/2 inch → Found by women practicing regular breast self-examination

1 inch → Found by women practicing occasional breast self-examination

1 ½ inch → Found by women untrained in breast self-examination

*Sizes are approximate.
Graphic courtesy of the National Cancer Institute and the Breast Health Program of New York.

Figure 2-1: Benefits of Regular Mammograms and Breast Examinations (The average size of tumor found with different types of screening)

the likelihood that some will anchor and nest in the blood vessels of another organ, creating metastases. The greater the probability of metastases, the lower the probability of cure.

Following this logic, the key to success in cancer management is to find cancer before it is invasive, or if invasive, as soon as possible before it METAS-TASIZES. Breast self-exams, physician breast exams, and mammography are intended to do just that. There seems to be little downside to knowing your body through self-exam, undergoing an annual physical with breast exam, and undergoing age-appropriate mammography. Dr. Scott had exactly the same thoughts when he ordered the mammogram for Jill. I could say much more, but this is truly an example where a picture is worth a thousand words (Figure 2-1).

The controversy surrounding breast cancer screening relates to the concept that a screening tool must be both sensitive and specific. Numerous observations challenge the SPECIFICITY and SENSITIVITY of breast cancer screenings in younger women. First, the density of the breast tissue of a young woman such as Jill decreases the sensitivity of both the mammogram and the exam. Also, exams in young, menstruating women are notoriously unreliable because so many changes in the breast are not specific to cancer. Finally, the chance of breast cancer in a 40-year-old woman is very low, just 1 in 1,000, leading to a very low index of suspicion. Combined, these issues lead to problems ranging from early cancers being neither visualized nor suspected to noncancerous changes creating misleading findings leading to unnecessary biopsies and anguish. Newer and better methods are needed to screen young, high-risk women, as is discussed later in this chapter.

Jill's exam was normal, and her mammogram abnormalities were at best merely suspicious given the difficulties of interpreting her young, dense breasts. The repeat mammogram involved a magnification of the suspicious area, which still was questionably a cancer. Examining this area on ultrasound left no doubt that waiting six months to repeat the breast imaging was not a safe alternative. A biopsy was needed to examine the mammary cells in this suspicious area of the breast. What the doctors failed to find on exam but found suspicious on imaging and worrisome on biopsy was our next discussion.

## Clinical Findings

The female breast changes dramatically with age. The flow of estrogen at puberty initiates the development of the breast, specifically the mammary tissue. The ebb and flow of sex hormones during menstrual cycles cause the breast to swell cyclically and become tender. Pregnancy produces further breast enlargement, which is fostered as long as lactation is stimulated by breastfeeding. The PERIMENOPAUSAL years are accompanied by the regression of mammary tissue and its replacement by fat. All of these changes are usually uniform and symmetrical. The hallmark of clinical breast disease is asymmetry, a visible or PALPABLE defect (clinical change) in one breast. Unfortunately, cancers that produce an asymmetrical defect of the breast are often large and advanced.

Findings of breast asymmetry—whether palpable breast deformity (lump, ridge), unilateral nipple dimpling or discharge, changes in the skin of the breast, or a lump in the armpit (AXILLA)—all warrant immediate medical evaluation (Figure 2-2). A woman who examines her breasts routinely will become familiar with the normal hormone-induced changes of her menstrual cycle and more sensitive to an asymmetrical or discrete defect as described here. A physician's exam benefits from the experience of having felt and seen diseased breasts but lacks the sensitivity of the woman who examines herself regularly.

Jill had been performing monthly breast self-examinations since she was 35. She was accustomed to breast enlargement and tenderness before her menses, but she had not noted anything unusual. Dr. Scott's annual exams had also been unremarkable, but there was obviously something there.

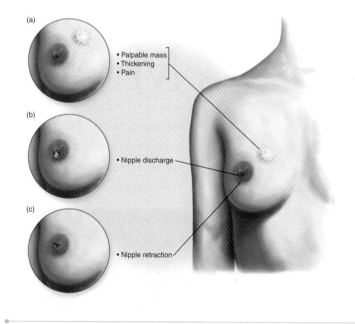

Figure 2-2: Breast Cancer: Possible Signs and Symptoms

# Breast Imaging:

The continued commitment to improve the early detection of breast cancer, especially in premenopausal women, has led to a rapid expansion of breast imaging techniques. Although mammography remains the gold standard among breast cancer screening methods, new technologies are challenging traditional radiographic imaging in sensitivity, specificity and cost effectiveness. Let's take a minute to review those methods currently approved for use in patients with, or suspected of having, breast cancer. They include: CAD (COMPUTER AIDED DETECTION) MAMMOGRAPHY; DIGITAL MAMMOGRAPHY; BREAST ULTRASONOGRAPHY; MRI (MAGNETIC RESONANCE IMAGING); AND PET (POSITRON EMISSION TOMOGRAPHY).

# Mammography—CAD and Digital:

Mammography, whether traditional, computer aided or digital, uses X-rays to produce an image of the breast. In traditional mammography, which came into common use in the early 1970s, the image is developed directly on film. In CAD mammography that film is scanned into a computer that uses special software to aid in the identification of abnormalities. In digital mammography the X-ray image is directly converted to an electronic image. The progress in mammography mirrors that of photography in general. Not many years ago our cameras created picture negatives that we had to have

Figure 2-3 A: Normal

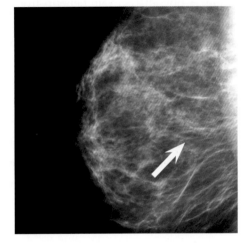

Figure 2-3 B: Micro Calcification (questionable DCIS)

Figure 2-3 C: Coarse Calcification (Benign)

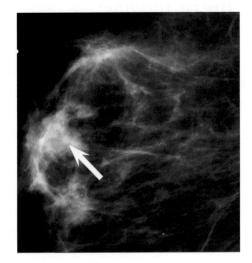

Figure 2-3 D: Stellate Lesion (questionable tumor)

developed. Then we had computers that allowed us to scan our developed images into a database. Today we mostly use digital cameras. Our photos may never exist in hard copy; they reside on our phones and computers and not in bulky photo albums subject to fading, tearing, wrinkling and being lost.

Uploading images to a digital database offers both the obvious as well as theoretical benefits. The images can be easily stored and retrieved, making review among experts, even at long distance, easy. Images can be adjusted (e.g., magnified, contrasted), thus enhancing subtle differences in contiguous tissues. Specialized software can be utilized to aid the radiologist's interpretation and thereby improve accuracy: both specificity and sensitivity. Finally, such improvements in accuracy permit lower doses of radiation to be used. Despite all these apparent benefits, only 10% or so of mammographies performed in the U.S. are currently digital. Why? Two reasons: It costs more, and studies conclusively proving the ultimate benefit—fewer deaths from breast cancer—have yet to be completed. One large randomized clinical trial, titled DMIST, did show significantly better screening accuracy for: women under age 50; women of any age with dense breasts; and women older than 50 but less than one year from last menses. Future efforts to improve mammography will continue to focus on refining the technology and improving how it is administered.

# Breast Ultrasonography:

The breast ultrasound or sonogram is an imaging technique that uses high frequency sound waves instead of penetrating X-rays to image the breast. The sound waves, too high a frequency to be heard, are directed into the breast tissue from a TRANSDUCER held against the skin of the breast. The sound waves bounce or reflect off the various tissues of the breast, (e.g., duct, lobule, fat, etc.) differently. The echoes of sound created by the reflections are received by the transducer and, via attached computer, translated into an image, the SONOGRAM. Ultrasonography is particularly useful in distinguishing a solid from a liquid structure, (e.g., a tumor from a cyst) and in identifying palpable abnormalities not seen on mammography. Ultrasonography is not used for routine breast cancer screening as it lacks sensitivity for microcalcifications, one of the earliest imaging findings detectable in DCIS and early invasive cancer.

# Magnetic Resonance Imaging (MRI):

Like Ultrasonography, MRI also images the breast without penetrating X-rays. The science behind MRI is a bit more complex to both explain and understand. Essentially, the breast is placed into a powerful electromagnetic field, which causes the tissues of the breast to vibrate or resonate. Like the differential echoes that are the basis of ultrasonography, the differential resonance is the basis of MRI. Once again, a computer translates the differential resonances into an anatomic image. Breast MRI is not recommended for routine breast cancer screening because of its lack of specificity: It does not distinguish between benign and malignant lesions of the breast. However, MRI's very high degree of sensitivity make it very valuable for high risk younger women with dense breasts, especially those with hereditary genetic predisposition.

# Positron Emission Tomography (PET):

Unlike the imaging techniques discussed thus far, PET is a physiologic or functional imaging technique as well as an anatomic one. Most body imaging tries to reveal anatomic changes that are the hallmark of disease, such as a fractured bone, pneumonia, or gallstones. Some imaging, referred to as NUCLEAR, uses Geiger counter type measurement of radioactive isotope accumulation in an organ to evaluate its function (e.g., thyroid scan). PET combines anatomic imaging with a CT scanner and functional imaging with a radioactive isotope to do both.

The body is comprised of cells, and all cells use the same fuel: sugar (glucose). Cancer cells take up more sugar per unit of time than normal cells. So researchers developed a technique whereby differential uptake of radioactive sugar could be both measured and correlated with an anatomic abnormality revealed on CT scan to deduce if that abnormality was benign or malignant. Thus PET may play a role in determining whether a breast abnormality is cancerous. However, since PET imaging is more accurate in detecting larger (>1 cm) and aggressive (invasive) tumors, it is more commonly used in staging and restaging cancer than in screening (to be discussed in Chapter 4).

Advances in the science and the technology of breast imaging are not isolated. They parallel those that are taking place in both the pathologic diagnosis and the treatment of breast cancer. Modern medicine continues to strive to develop objective, verifiable and reproducible criteria upon which all care can be based. The image of a radiologist squinting at a view-box holding a hard copy mammogram is being replaced by that of a radiologist manipulating digital images on a computer monitor, assisted by software. The image of the pathologist peering through the microscope lens trying to determine if the scant cells before his/her eyes are abnormal enough to call cancer is being replaced by a computer assisted measurement of the protein content of thousands of cells. The image of the oncologist deep in thought with furrowed brow trying to decide if the patient across the consult desk needs chemotherapy in addition to five years of an anti-estrogen pill is being replaced by a validated 21-gene tumor profile that predicts outcome based on therapy. This is the modern era of medicine, more science than art, as Jill and Gregg were now beginning to realize.

As I explained the limitations of breast screening in young women, Jill almost felt fortunate that the radiologist detected an abnormality. She now understood why annual mammography is not recommended until women reach the age of 40 years and why it remains controversial until women reach the age of 50 years. She also understood that, for close relatives of breast cancer patients, their screening should begin 10 years younger than the age of their relative at diagnosis. This meant that her daughter Amy should undergo her first screening at age 27. That was a scary thought. I assured both Jill and Greg that in 20 years better screening tools, both genetic and radiographic, would surely be available. This seemed like a good time to discuss the genetic testing for breast cancer that is available today.

## Hereditary Breast Cancer and Genetic Testing

Was there a test that could have predicted Jill's breast cancer? If Jill underwent the testing now and it proved that she was predisposed to breast cancer, would it change her choice of treatment? If Jill tested positive, should she test Amy?

If genetic events govern a cell's behavior, then genetic changes must be present before a cell transforms. However, scientists are still working to understand what changes occur among the thousands of genes in each cell, leading that cell to cancer. If a cell has 40,000 genes and just 1% of those genes mutated to confer on that cell a cancerous behavior, then 400 mutated genes would be present. If only 40 gene mutations could lead to cancer, then you would have to find 40 abnormal genes among 40,000 normal ones. Genetic testing for cancer is the ultimate needle in the haystack search. Amazingly, sometimes the detective work pays off.

After many years of scientists searching for the elusive breast cancer gene, in September 1994 the Journal *Science* announced the cloning of BRCA-1 (located on chromosome 17). This report linked mutations in the gene with breast and ovarian cancer in a handful of families. Later in the same month, a second breast cancer gene, BRCA-2, was identified in the long arm of chromosome 13. It is believed that BRCA-1 and BRCA-2 are responsible for most hereditary breast cancers. However, hereditary breast cancer is believed to account for only 5% to 10% of all breast cancer cases, as was discussed in Chapter 1.

One in every 200 women in the United States is thought to carry a defective BRCA-1 or BRCA-2 gene. The lifetime risk of developing breast cancer in a patient with BRCA-1 or BRCA-2 is 85% (normal lifetime risk = 12%). There is a 44% risk of developing ovarian cancer in patients who test positive for BRCA-1. The ovarian cancer risk of BRCA-2 is lower. As many as 30% of the women diagnosed with breast cancer before the age of 40 may be carriers of these mutations or other mutations yet to be identified.

Tests for both BRCA-1 and BRCA-2 are commercially available. Genetic counseling is the most important part of genetic screening, and in most major testing centers more than 50% of patients who are counseled refuse testing.

## Genetic counseling includes:

1. INFORMED CONSENT
2. Counseling regarding the risk of cancer
3. The availability of therapy for cancer
4. Referral back to the physician once testing has been complete
5. Post-test counseling

The individuals at high risk for the breast/ovarian cancer syndrome include those people who have two first-degree relatives (sibling, parent, child) with breast and/or ovarian cancer or three second- or third-degree relatives with breast and/or ovarian cancer. There is some suggestion that younger patients with breast cancer should be tested even without a significant family history because of their higher chances of carrying the BRCA-1 and BRCA-2 genes. Although this has not been conclusively proven, it does enable doctors to relax the testing criteria for the younger patient (under age 40 years) population. It is important to note that the risk factors for hereditary breast cancer are more specific than the general risk factors for all breast cancers.

General risk factors are issues in a woman's personal medical history that may predispose her to the acquired genetic mutations that give rise to breast cancer (Table 2-1). Researchers have developed mathematical models that quantify an individual's lifetime breast cancer risk as compared to the general population of age-matched controls. These computer programs that use personal and family history to estimate a woman's chance of developing breast cancer are often referred to as the GAIL MODEL, as this was the first such program to be readily available to the community of breast cancer patients and caregivers. These programs are not validated for women with a history of DCIS, LCIS, or those who are known to be BRCA-1 or BRCA-2 carriers.

- Personal history of breast cancer
- Family history of breast cancer, especially in first-degree relatives
- Atypical ductal or lobular hyperplasia
- Early first menses, late menopause
- Late first pregnancy / no pregnancy
- Exogenous estrogens (external patches, pill)
- Radiation that has involved the breast
- Family member who is BRCA positive

Table 2-1: Breast Cancer Risk Factors

As discussed in Chapter 1, all cancer is, in the final analysis, a genetic disease. Whether the cancer is the result of a hereditary mutation such as BRCA-1 or sequential acquired mutations, gene mutations are the root cause of cellular transformation. Changes in a woman's genome precede the transformation of a normal mammary cell to an adenocarcinoma. Changes in the proteins, the design of which are governed by those genes, also precede carcinogenesis. A new field of research has evolved to study the sequential changes of the gene and protein composition of mammary cancer cells, with hopes that a predictive pattern of change will be observed. If such observations are successful, then it may be possible to diagnose women before the completion of carcinogenesis. These new fields of gene and protein research are called, respectively, GENOMICS and PROTEINOMICS. The analysis of likely gene and protein predictors is called MICROARRAY TESTING. In the not too distant future, we may be able to create a cancer fingerprint, a unique genetic and protein signature or bar code that identifies a cancer in development, before clinical detection and before invasion. Women found to have a high-risk gene/protein fingerprint may be treated before their cancer develops or be monitored for further mutations (Figure 2-4). Genomic and proteinomic analysis may not yet be ready for prime time as a breast cancer screening tool, but they have already become a mainstream tool in the determination of treatment, as we'll see in Chapter 4.

As both a daughter and the mother of a daughter, Jill decided to undergo genetic testing and counseling. Unfortunately, the testing would take two weeks to complete. Jill and Greg dreaded the thought of two more weeks of waiting. The genetic testing was important, as it would impact both her mother and daughter, but, would it change Jill and Greg's choice and timing of surgery? We decided to continue our discussions about her biopsy and the possible treatments that would still be needed.

Figure 2-4: Relationship of Mutational Events to Carcinogenesis

# Evaluation of the Breast Lump

A woman or man with a lump or defect in the breast found on self-exam, physician exam, and/or confirmed on breast imaging (mammogram or ultrasound) requires prompt medical attention. Fortunately, not every lump or defect in the breast is cancer. Unfortunately, in many instances, the only way to be sure there is cancer is to remove the defect and view the cells under a microscope. Most often, after exam and a review of the mammogram and ultrasound, the physician will perform or request a biopsy. Biopsies range from FINE-NEEDLE ASPIRATION performed in the office to surgical removal of the lump in an outpatient surgery center.

When a lump is palpated or a solid defect is observed on imaging, a needle biopsy can be performed. When a fine-needle aspiration or needle biopsy is performed, the cells that comprise the defect or lump will be aspirated (sucked out) and viewed under the microscope to determine whether the cellular material is of mammary origin (not merely blood and/or fat) and whether those cells are cancerous.

Sometimes a larger needle is used to remove a slender core of breast tissue (the diameter of lead in a lead pencil). This is called a CORE BIOPSY. Specialized radiographic imaging equipment is sometimes used to facilitate the biopsy, a procedure referred to as a STEREOTACTIC BREAST BIOPSY. Specialized biopsy devices are also employed, such as a MAMMOTOME. Other times, a piece of the defect will be cut out (INCISIONAL BIOPSY) or the entire lump will be removed (EXCISIONAL BIOPSY). (Figure 2-5 A, B, C, D) Regardless of the technology used, the microscopic or pathologic review will determine whether cancer cells are present and whether they are confined to the duct space or invading through the duct wall.

Most often, the surgeon will attempt to remove the entire defect or abnormality of the breast by performing an excisional biopsy, often referred to as a LUMPECTOMY. This is also necessary when a solid lump is not appreciated but microcalcifications are observed. The pathologic and microscopic review of an excisional biopsy must not only determine whether the cells present are cancerous and invasive but also whether all of the cancer cells have been removed. The only way to know whether all of the cancer cells are removed is to see a halo or rim of normal cells surrounding the entire cancer

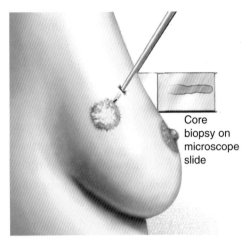

Cells on
microscope
slide

Core
biopsy on
microscope
slide

Figure 2-5 A: Fine Needle Aspiration

Figure 2-5 B: Core Biopsy

Wedge of
abnormal
breast tissue

Excised
breast
lump

Figure 2-5 C: Incisional Biopsy

Figure 2-5 D: Excisional Biopsy

lump. This halo of normal cells surrounding the diseased cells is referred to as the MARGIN. Margins will be identified as clean (uninvolved with cancer) or dirty (cancer cells extend to the edge of the specimen). A clean margin will be further categorized by the width of the halo by either measurement (e.g., 1 mm margin) or narrative (close margin). Margins are discussed in more detail later as they relate to treatment.

Regardless of the type of biopsy, this is the critical step in defining the cancer process. **Cancer can be confirmed only by a pathologist's review of an appropriate specimen under a microscope.** All of the X-rays and exams preceding the biopsy can only suggest or raise the suspicion of cancer. Only after a biopsy can the pronouncement "you have cancer" be made. After that, all medical efforts are directed at planning the cancer treatment. The finding of invasive cancer adds a layer of complexity to the treatment planning, as we will see in the following chapters.

Jill underwent a stereotactic biopsy, which to the surprise of the radiologist and surgeon not only revealed DCIS but also an area of invasive cancer. The cancer was not completely removed. A small piece of the tumor, or core biopsy, was taken for analysis to help Jill and Greg and the doctors select the most appropriate surgical option. Options are both a blessing and a curse, especially when they produce equal results. "Just tell me what I need to do," or "What would you do?" or "What would you recommend to your wife or mother?" are common questions. How could patients possibly decide when they feel so overwhelmed and so poorly informed? Jill and Greg had decisions to make, but first they needed to understand that surgery was not just about removing the lump of cancerous mammary tissue.

# Chapter Three

# Breast Cancer Treatment: History, Science, Practice

## Noninvasive Versus Invasive

Unfortunately, many cancers are not found when they remain confined to the duct, but only after there has been invasion through the duct wall. I had explained to Jill and Greg that when there is invasion there is a risk that the cancer has not only infiltrated surrounding mammary tissue but also invaded the walls of nearby blood vessels, thereby gaining access to the circulation and other organs. One of the greatest challenges of medical science is to develop strategies to find and destroy rogue cancer cells circulating in the bloodstream of the patient with newly diagnosed invasive breast cancer.

In many patients with invasive breast cancer, the challenge of finding rogue cancer cells in the circulation is analogous to finding a needle in a haystack. As you recall from Chapter 1, cells grow by doubling. That rogue cancer cell that survives downstream will become two, those two will become four, etc. Cells are microscopic: 1,000 can fit in a grain of sand, and 25,000 can fit on the head of a pin (Figure 3-1). None of our current diagnostic studies—neither laboratory tests nor CT, MRI, and PET scans—can detect cancer at that microscopic level.

Physicians and patients are in the uncomfortable position of knowing that cancer cells may be loose in the circulation without having any proof. Any observation that might predict the probability of cancer cell contamination outside the breast is critical to planning the treatment of the breast cancer patient. The patient's age, the size of the tumor, the tumor cell's sensitivity to estrogen, and the presence of increased amounts of the gene HER-2/NEU (these features

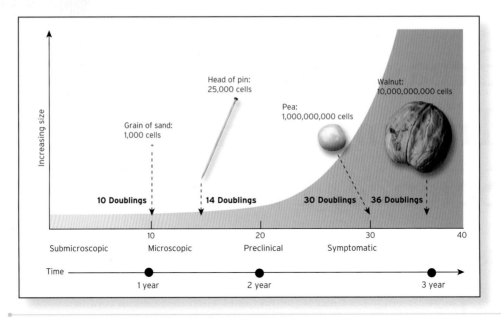

Figure 3-1: Exponential Growth of Cancer Cells

will be discussed in more depth in future chapters) have all demonstrated predictive value, but the presence of cancer cells within the LYMPH NODES of the breast is the single most important factor in predicting breast cancer cell spread outside of the breast.

## Evaluation of the Lymph Nodes

I ask patients like Jill and Greg to try to stay focused as I explain the LYMPHATIC SYSTEM and the need to evaluate the lymph nodes draining the area of the breast in which the tumor was found. They need to understand that the presence or absence of lymph node contamination is the single most predictive finding regarding relapse and cure. I begin by explaining the relationship between lymph and blood.

Another type of blood channel runs alongside the blood vessels in the breast and throughout the body. These are called lymph channels. Lymph and blood are related. Blood is composed of RED BLOOD CELLS, WHITE BLOOD CELLS, and PLATELETS, suspended in a fluid called PLASMA. The red blood cells carry oxygen to every living cell in the body. The white blood cells are survey-and-destroy foreign invaders (bacteria, viruses, etc.). The platelets are plug holes in traumatized blood vessels to prevent bleeding. Although all three types of cells circulate in blood vessels, only white blood cells circulate in the lymph system. If we think of the blood as nourishing all of the living cells of our body with oxygen and glucose (sugar), we might think of the lymph as washing every living cell, washing out bacteria, viruses, and anything foreign to our body that might infect or injure it. With lymph channels flowing side by side with blood vessels, if a root or tentacle of tumor has invaded through the duct wall and into the wall of an underlying blood vessel, most likely it has also invaded through a lymph channel (Figure 3-2).

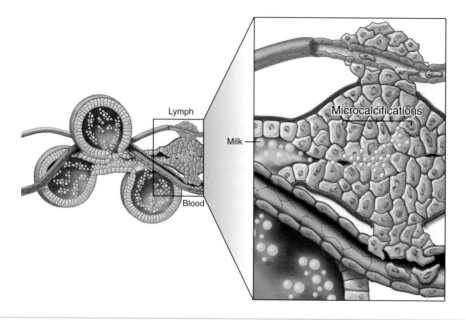

Figure 3-2: Vascular and Lymphatic Invasion

Unlike the blood, which flows uninterrupted from organ to organ delivering oxygen and nutrients to each cell it touches, the lymph is filtered between organs by structures called lymph nodes. When the white blood cells in the lymph have surrounded bacteria or viruses, these microbes are filtered out by the lymph node, where special killing cells destroy the foreign invaders, preventing further spread. Unfortunately, cancer cells originate (mutate) from our own cells. Despite their sometimes bizarre appearance and aggressive behavior as well as their potential to harm the body, they still appear human to the IMMUNE SYSTEM. Therefore, the cancer cells are not recognized as foreign invaders, and they are not destroyed. They are, however, trapped in

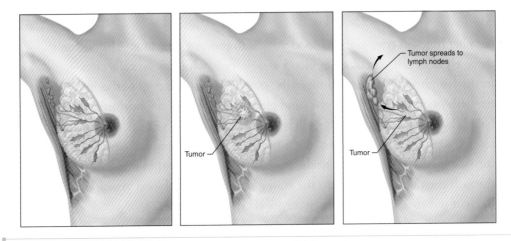

Tumor spreads to lymph nodes

Tumor

Tumor

Figure 3-3: Breast Cancer Evolution from Benign to Nodal Spread

the lymph node. If they are living but are trapped, they will multiply, and a nest will grow (Figure 3-3).

This is critical knowledge for doctors who are managing breast cancer patients. The lymph nodes are a window into the circulatory system and help doctors understand the potential risk for cancer spread. A pinhead-size cluster of cancer cells that would have escaped detection by physical examination, laboratory testing, and radiographic imaging anywhere else in the body can be found in a lymph node when the node is examined under a microscope. If a lymph node is found to be contaminated by a nest of cancer cells, then the cancer likely did not only invade the lymph channel but also the neighboring blood vessel. Lymph involvement confirms that despite removing the cancerous tumor, there may still be microscopic cancer cells contaminating the body. These are referred to as MICROMETASTASES. The relationship between node contamination and risk of micrometastases is linear: The greater the extent of lymph node involvement, the greater the risk of systemic contamination.

The distinction between noninvasive and invasive cancer, the predictive value of lymph node involvement, and the increasing understanding of the natural history of breast cancer have led to an evolution in doctors' strategies in diagnosing and managing a breast compromised by cancer. Having gotten this far with my patients, such as Jill and Greg, the next step is to explain the different surgical options. I usually begin this discussion by providing some historical background.

# Evolution of Breast Cancer Management

Our understanding of cancer has changed quite a bit over the past century. It was over 100 years ago that the first effective breast cancer treatments were published. At that time, the only treatment was surgery, formulated on the notion that cancer was a manifestation of a diseased organ. The only way to eradicate the disease was by radical surgery to remove the entire organ with its blood supply and lymph drainage.

The doctors of the late 19th and early 20th centuries believed that cancer would spread from the diseased organ to the draining lymph nodes and only then to other organs. Therefore, the cancer could be stopped by removing, resecting, or dissecting out all of the lymph nodes that drain the cancerous organ. The majority of the nodes that drain the breast are located under the arm in the armpit, which is anatomically called the AXILLA; hence, the surgery to remove all the lymph nodes (approximately 40) from the axilla is called a COMPLETE AXILLARY NODE DISSECTION.

For nearly 100 years, breast cancer patients not only underwent complete axillary node dissection, but doctors also removed the entire breast as well as the muscles beneath the breast and the blood vessels supplying the area. This was called a RADICAL MASTECTOMY. The radical mastectomy with its requisite complete axillary node dissection was not only quite deforming but also it was associated with late COMPLICATIONS, the most serious of which was IPSILATERAL or same-side arm LYMPHEDEMA. Lymphedema is a swelling of the arm after its draining axillary lymph nodes and veins have been injured by surgery and/or radiation. The arm may swell three to four times normal size, causing pain and restricting motion. The lymphedematous arm is also more susceptible to infections, which is why doctors recommend that neither blood draw nor blood pressure monitoring be performed on it.

During the past 30 to 40 years of cancer research, scientists began to realize that the cancer problem is not what you can see with the unaided eye, not merely a local or even a regional problem of an organ and its draining lymph nodes. Rather breast cancer, like all organ cancer, is a total body or SYSTEMIC disease. The cancer cells gain access to the entire circulatory system and can nest microscopically and invisibly anywhere in the body. Curing cancer was less related to the extent of breast surgery and more related to the ability of medical science to develop treatments that would destroy the breast cancer cells at large in the body.

By the last quarter of the 20th century, radical mastectomies and complete axillary lymph node dissections had become inconsistent with the new systemic theory of cancer, which stated that a cancer's dissemination into the blood circulation develops not after lymph node spread but rather simultaneously with lymphatic involvement.

Understanding the differences between invasive and noninvasive cancer as well as the emerging systemic theory of cancer helped doctors realize that they could limit the extent of breast surgery without compromising a cure. Incorporating scientific theory into clinical practice led to the less deforming MODIFIED RADICAL MASTECTOMY which preserved the pectoralis muscle and the higher level nodes. More recently, the desire to preserve the breast has resulted in further reductions in the extent of breast surgery, leading to the SIMPLE MASTECTOMY, BREAST-CONSERVATION SURGERY (also called PARTIAL MASTECTOMY), SEGMENTAL MASTECTOMY, and LUMPECTOMY. These organ-sparing or breast-conserving surgeries, when complemented by breast irradiation to sterilize the remaining mammary tissue, have proven equal in effectiveness to the more radical surgical approaches for nearly 90% of breast cancer patients. Preserving the breast without compromising cure has made the lumpectomy the procedure of choice for the majority of breast cancer patients (Figure 3-4).

In conjunction with reductions in breast surgery, researchers began advocating smaller lymph node samplings. They advised taking only the most likely contaminated and accessible nodes, approximately 10 on average, in a procedure called AXILLARY SAMPLING. Even more recently, doctors have recognized that lymph drainage coming from an area of the breast typically flows to one particular lymph node as the first in a chain to receive that lymph drainage. That first lymph node in the chain to receive drainage from the area of the breast lump is called the SENTINEL LYMPH NODE. Research now demonstrates that adequate lymph node evaluation can be achieved by injecting dye within the location of the breast lump (tumor), watching over 30 minutes to see which lymph node is the first to accept the dye (LYMPHOSCINTIGRAPHY), and then removing that sentinel lymph node

(SENTINEL NODE BIOPSY) (Figure 3-5). If the sentinel node is free of cancer, no further lymph node surgery is required.

When I read or hear comments suggesting that little progress has been made in the management of breast cancer, I am quick to respond that in the past 30 years the surgical management of breast cancer has been reduced from the radical mastectomy, with complete axillary dissection, to the mere removal of a lump and a single lymph node.

Figure 3-4:
Breast Surgery Options

Radical Mastectomy

Modified
radical mastectomy

Quadrantectomy

Lumpectomy

Jill was clearly a candidate for breast-conservation surgery, but her eligibility was just one factor to consider in her decision-making process. Because breast conservation required radiation, she and Greg needed to know more about radiation treatment.

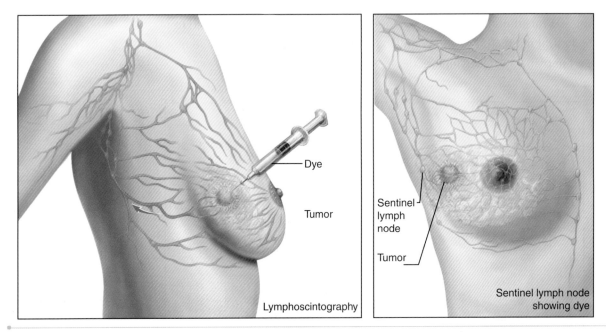

Dye

Tumor

Lymphoscintography

Sentinel lymph node

Tumor

Sentinel lymph node showing dye

Figure 3-5: Sentinel Node Evaluation

# Role of Radiation Therapy in Locoregional Disease

Figure 3-6: Radiant Energy

I explained to Jill and Greg that before they could understand the role radiation would play in her cure, they needed to understand what therapeutic radiation is.

Picture a pebble being tossed into a pond and the wave-like ripples that simultaneously emerge in all directions from the point of impact. Now with that picture in mind, imagine a lit candle afloat in the middle of the pond with its light radiating in all directions. Like the ripples in the water after a pebble toss, radiant energy also emanates in omnidirectional waves from its source, except that these waves are invisible. Science refers to that visible light as RADIANT ENERGY (Figure 3-6).

Radiant energy is classified by the distance between the waves, referred to as WAVELENGTHS. Wavelengths vary greatly, ranging from wider than a million meters to as narrow as one billionth of a meter. This mind-boggling range of radiant energy wavelengths makes up the ELECTROMAGNETIC SPECTRUM. The shortest wavelengths are those that produce therapeutic radiation. The longest wavelengths are those associated with electricity. In between these extremes, as we move from short to long in the electromagnetic spectrum, are diagnostic X-rays; ultraviolet light; visible light; infrared light; microwaves; radar; and television, radio, and communication frequencies (Figure 3-7).

Therapeutic radiation, also called GAMMA RADIATION, refers to the clinical use of radiant energy emitted by radioactive substances housed in a 2-ton machine called a LINEAR ACCELERATOR. Like the ultraviolet radiant energy from the sun that can affect skin by damaging cells on the skin surface, gamma radiation can penetrate below the skin, damaging cells internally. Computers and special equipment called COLLUMNATORS permit the gamma rays to be focused and contoured to a particular structure of the body such as

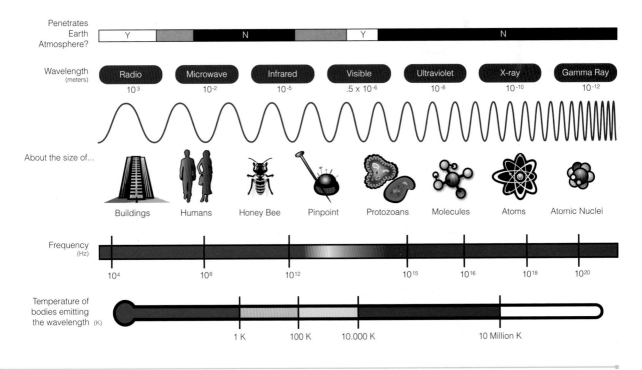

Figure 3-7: Electromagnetic Spectrum

the breast. At a high enough exposure to gamma radiation, cells may not only be injured but also killed. Research has revealed that there is a narrow range or threshold dose of gamma radiation that, when delivered repeatedly (each dose called a FRACTION) to cancer cells, will kill the cancer cells without killing the surrounding normal cells. Therapeutic radiation exploits this research to develop treatment strategies for different cancer problems. Returning to our sun-bathing analogy, too much sun exposure at one time will cause skin injury (sun-burn) but daily brief exposures result in controlled tanning. Similarly, controlled gamma radiation exposure can produce desired results.

Therapeutic radiation may play a variety of roles in the treatment of breast cancer. Most commonly, it is used to sterilize a breast of possible residual microscopic cancer cell contamination after a cancerous tumor has been surgically removed, thus permitting preservation of the breast (breast-conservation surgery therapy). Even when the breast has been removed, radiation treatments may be recommended for the skin of the chest and the remaining axillary lymph nodes if the cancerous tumor was very large (>5 cm) or if multiple lymph nodes (>3) were found to be contaminated. Controversy continues regarding radiation's role in large tumors (3–5 cm), contaminated nodes (3 or fewer), close margins and multifocal invasive disease. Finally, radiation treatments may be helpful in controlling symptoms from nests of breast cancer cells that may have grown in other parts of the body (metastases), especially in the bone.

Novel research in therapeutic radiation is now developing new technologies to improve external radiation targeting, implant radioactive seeds, and inject targeted radioactive molecules. One of theses new radiation technologies is often referred to as PARTIAL BREAST IRRADIATION (MAMOSITE), a targeted breast radiation therapy. Therapeutic radiation remains a critical component of breast cancer treatment planning, as explained in future chapters.

# Management of the Breast (Locoregional Therapy)

Jill and Greg had now learned about the evaluation of the breast. They understood why the lymph nodes are important and how doctors can minimize the complications from breast and lymph node surgery by using breast conservation approaches, limited lymph node sampling, and sentinel node analysis. They also understood the relationship between the extent of node involvement and the risk of metastases. Now I wanted to turn their attention to how ONCOLOGISTS integrate these treatments.

The local (breast) and regional (lymph nodes, chest wall) treatment options for breast cancer are numerous. Many factors should be considered when selecting treatment for this disease. Physician and patient preferences, patient age and anatomy, tumor characteristics (including size, location, and pathology), genetic profiling, and patient and family history are all important considerations. Although management of the involved breast and the uninvolved breast and the method of lymph node evaluation remain individually specific, as is discussed later, some general comments about locoregional therapy are relevant here.

If the biopsy confirms cancer, but it is confined to the duct space (DCIS), then removing it, in theory, cures the cancer. However, removal or excision must be complete. To assure complete excision, the pathologist evaluates tissue along the edge or cut margin of the excised lump of DCIS to make sure that there is normal mammary tissue surrounding the entire focus of DCIS. If DCIS is found on any surface of the excised lump, it is referred to as a contaminated margin and further surgery (RE-EXCISION) will likely be needed to achieve complete tumor removal (Figure 3-8).

Visualize a peach that you halved, removed the pit, then bit into only to find some pit-like grit in your mouth. The pit was removed and to the eye the peach half looked ready to eat, but now you have to take a spoon and remove some more—that's re-excision. If the breast is small or the cancer extensive, re-excision may not be feasible.

However, even when all margins are free of cancer cell contamination, confirming that the cancerous tumor has been completely removed, a problem exists: research has revealed that precancerous changes may reside in other parts of the same breast. There could be atypical hyperplasia or even DCIS that was not yet visible on mammogram or palpable on exam. Precancerous areas within other parts of the same breast if not identified and not treated, could emerge later as invasive disease. Thus, not only do doctors have to remove

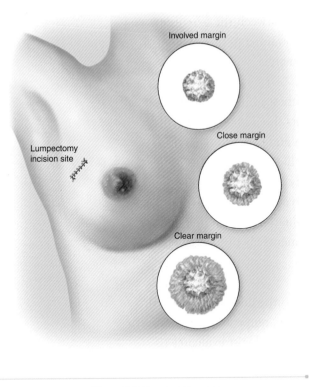

Involved margin

Close margin

Lumpectomy
incision site

Clear margin

Figure 3-8: Surgical Margins

the area of DCIS in its entirety, but they also need to treat the remaining mammary tissue of the diseased breast. The finding of DCIS in one part of the breast identifies cancer risk throughout the breast.

Currently, there are two standard ways to treat a breast with completely excised, clear margin, DCIS. One way is to remove the breast in its entirety (SIMPLE MASTECTOMY). The other way is to use high energy in the form of EXTERNAL BEAM RADIATION THERAPY to sterilize the remaining mammary tissue after the lump is completely removed by breast-conservation surgery. In patients with DCIS, doctors are not worried about spread throughout the body because, as long as the cancer is confined to the duct space, there is no risk of spread through blood or lymph. Therefore, lymph nodes are not removed for pathologic review.

More than 90% of patients with DCIS can choose the option of breast-conserving surgery, confident that breast preservation will not compromise the chance of cure. Mastectomy is preferred in a minority of patients: those in whom DCIS is extensive, those where DCIS location prevents a good cosmetic outcome, and those with severe fibrocystic disease which compromises future screening.

Regardless of the choice of management of the diseased breast, there remains a concern of future cancer in the uninvolved breast. Annual mammography and a physician exam as well as monthly self-exams are therefore a must. As discussed in Chapter 2, molecular testing and genetic testing to assess risk of breast cancer are becoming available to allow those women at very high risk to choose preventative or PROPHYLACTIC bilateral mastectomy. Recently, drug treatment strategies have been developed to prevent new breast cancers in both the involved and uninvolved breast (discussed in Chapter 6).

If the biopsy confirms an invasive ductal carcinoma, as in Jill's, the situation is similar to the one I just discussed. The entire breast remains at risk and must be treated even if the tumor has been removed and a clear margin confirmed. Again, the option is to remove the breast in its entirety or to sterilize it with radiation, both of which have been found to be equally effective in the great majority of women. However, in the patient with invasive cancer, something else still needs to be done. The lymph nodes that filter the breast's lymph circulation may hold clues to the risk that this cancer has gained access to the blood circulation. Those lymph nodes are under the arm (armpit or axilla) and need to be evaluated. Simple breast management will not be adequate here. The surgical options in a patient with invasive cancer must include axillary sampling or sentinel node evaluation.

Jill and Greg clearly understood the surgical options. She was an appropriate surgical candidate for breast conservation and was not bothered by the need for future radiation treatment. Alternatively, she could have the breast removed and undergo an immediate breast reconstruction. However, Jill and Greg remained concerned about Jill being genetically predisposed to breast cancer as she was so young. Jill was seriously considering having a bilateral mastectomy followed by immediate bilateral breast reconstruction. The meeting that was scheduled with the reconstructive surgeon in the morning would help them finalize their decision.

# Reconstructive Surgery

Breast reconstruction has become part and parcel the discussion of local breast management. The breast surgeon and reconstructive surgeon work closely to optimize the surgery technically and logistically. Once a patient's general health is assessed, the reconstructive surgeon will explain which options are most appropriate based on age, anatomy, tissue quality, and goals. Jill was fortunate, as she had no issues in her medical history that might complicate reconstruction. She had no serious medical problems. She was not obese and she did not smoke. Jill, Greg, and the reconstructive surgeon had a frank discussion of options as well as the risks and limitations of each. She also understood that general anesthesia was required for each procedure.

Chest muscles

Implant

Saline

Expander

Port

Figure 3-9: Expanded Implant

Jill seemed reassured that if she chose mastectomy, the currently available techniques and devices would make it possible for the surgeon to create a breast that would come close in form and appearance to her natural breast, it would replace. She also understood that reconstruction could be done immediately, during the same surgery as the mastectomy. She could wake up in the recovery room with a breast mound in place, never having the experience of seeing herself with no breast at all. She also understood that this was not a simple procedure; multiple surgeries would be needed to achieve a natural-appearing breast.

Despite the obvious benefits of immediate reconstruction, Jill knew there were legitimate reasons to wait. There were so many decisions to make. Was she prepared to also make the necessary decisions regarding her reconstruction now? She knew that postoperative complications of wound healing, bleeding, and infection could delay SYSTEMIC THERAPY. Even if systemic therapy was not delayed, was she prepared for the postoperative pain and the anticipated symptoms of healing?

Jill was able to summarize her options as two: an IMPLANT placed below the pectoralis muscle of the chest wall, or a full-thickness transplant of abdominal skin, fat, and muscle placed over the chest wall, called a TRAM flap (Transplanted Rectus Abdominus Muscle). A similar full thickness transplant of the latissimus muscle was also an alternative. The implant seemed easier. A noninflated plastic bag would be inserted under the pectoralis muscle after the mastectomy and gradually filled with saline over the subsequent weeks. Once the bag held enough saline and had stretched the muscle and skin to the size of her natural breast, the saline bag would be removed and a full-size implant inserted in its place (Figure 3-9). The alternative was a transplanted flap of skin and muscle from Jill's abdomen. The full-thickness flap from her abdomen would likely cause more pain, as the abdominal wound represents a second surgery; however, it would offer a more natural feel, as only living tissue would make up her new breast. She was intrigued that a flap of skin, fat, and muscle could be removed from her abdomen but remain connected to its blood vessels and nerves as it was turned upside down to make the breast (Figure 3-10). If she chose to have both breasts removed, this was definitely the better option as far as she and Greg were concerned. Jill and Greg were also aware, from their on-line research, that there was a great deal of research in new breast reconstruction procedures like the Free TRAM Flap, but felt comfortable with the choices presented by her surgeon.

Jill and Greg were clear that regardless of the extent of surgery, her hospitalization was unlikely to be less than two or more than five days. She understood that she might go home with a surgical drain, which removes excess blood and fluid from the wound. She knew that the drain and stitches would likely be out in 10 days, but it could take six weeks before she was completely recovered. Although scars would heal and fade over time, normal sensation would never be completely restored.

Jill and Greg were satisfied. They had reached a decision. All of their questions had been answered. The following week she would undergo the following surgeries: a right simple mastectomy to remove the cancer and the involved breast, a right axillary sentinel node biopsy to evaluate for node contamination by the invasive cancer, a left simple mastectomy to prevent a future left breast cancer, and bilateral breast reconstruction with a TRAM procedure. I told her I would visit her in the hospital before her discharge to review the final pathology of the breast and nodes. I told Greg I would call him and let him know when I would stop by the hospital room so that he could be there. They were still a bit uneasy knowing that, until the final pathology was reviewed, we could not discuss whether or what kind of systemic therapy might be needed.

Figure 3-10: TRAM Reconstruction

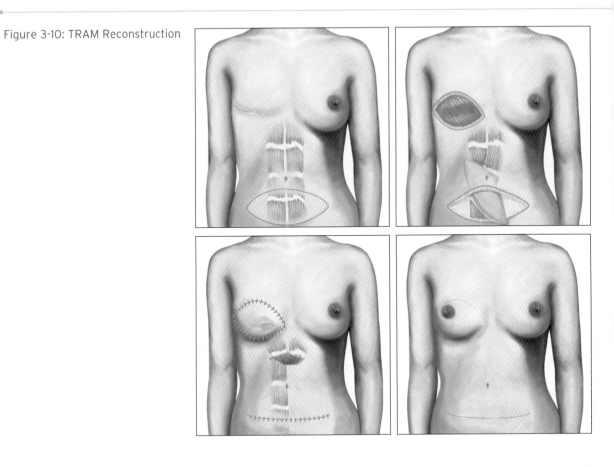

# SECTION 2

# After the Surgery

## Introduction

This section demystifies the postoperative return visit. We follow along with Jill and Greg as the pathology findings are organized into a quantifiable database referred to as STAGING. We review the relationship between STAGE and probability of cure. We then discuss the different types of postoperative treatments that can be used to improve the probability of cure. We review how research has improved the outcome for breast cancer patients as well as how ongoing CLINICAL TRIALS allow patients to gain access to new treatments. We try to make sense of the myriad of measurements used to assess the benefits of these systemic interventions. Let us return to Jill and Greg at their first postoperative visit to the office.

# Chapter Four

# Systemic Treatment Planning

Jill tolerated surgery well, without complication, leaving the hospital on the third postoperative day and before the final pathology report was available. I arranged for Jill and Greg to come by the office the following week to discuss the findings and their implications for further treatment. Unfortunately, although the breast tumor was found to be quite small (just over one centimeter), the sentinel lymph node was contaminated. The sentinel node was found to have a small cluster of cancer within it, requiring the surgeon to sample some additional lymph nodes. Fortunately, these additional nodes were not contaminated by the cancer. As I sat down with Jill and Greg to review the final pathology reports, they asked familiar questions: Is it good or bad? Did we catch it early? The root of these questions is this: Will I be cured? Fortunately for Jill, as for the majority of breast cancer patients, the answer is YES. Unfortunately, cure does not come without a cost, as the great majority of breast cancer patients must undergo systemic therapy after their breast and axillary lymph node surgery.

## Staging and Grading

It was time for the most difficult job I have as an oncologist: to explain to the patient that although the surgeon said "I got it all," what the surgeon meant to say was "I removed all of the cancer I could see." The critical distinction: Microscopic cancer may still reside in the body. No matter how positively I try to present the pathology findings, when the probability of cure is not 100%—and it usually is not—a cloud of gloom hangs over the discussion. Jill's chances of cure were excellent but not 100%, so I placed a box of tissues on my desk and emotionally prepared for our discussion.

ONCOLOGY in its essence is a discipline of medical science. In a scientific discipline, theory is tested by experiment, and success is measured quantitatively. In order to quantify the probability of cure or, inversely, the risk of cancer relapse, the oncologist must weigh the evidence that is available. The evidence is to be found in the pathology reports, laboratory tests, and imaging studies, but it must be organized in a meaningful and comparative way. The oncologic medical community responded to this need by standardizing a system for quantifying cancer, both the extent of disease and the characteristics that determine the risk of relapse and the probability of cure. Although it is the physician's desire to comfort and provide hope, there is no escaping an objective review of data with a patient and his/her family before they can provide an INFORMED CONSENT to undergo treatment.

Information gathered about the breast tumor pathology, the lymph node pathology, the radiographic imaging, and the laboratory data comprise the database. The database is organized to quantify or grade[2] the amount of disease locally within the breast, regionally within the lymph nodes, and systemically within other organs. This system of cancer measurement is referred to as cancer STAGING and addresses each area of disease as follows: the breast malignant growth or tumor (tumor = T) regarding its size, extent, and location (graded 1 to 4); the lymph nodes (nodes = N) regarding number, character, and location (graded 0 to 3); and evidence of other organ spread or metastases (metastases = M), either there is or there is not (graded 1 or 0). This is called the TNM STAGING SYSTEM (Table 4-1). The least amount of invasive cancer would be represented by a very small tumor (T1), without lymph node involvement (N0), and without spread to other organs (M0), or (T1 N0 M0). The worst scenario would be any cancer that had already spread to other organs of the body (T-any, N-any, M1). Staging allows doctors to categorize patients with similar cancer characteristics, thereby helping to predict outcomes and permitting treatment stratification based on risk. Stage I cancers are very small (less than 2 cm) and have no proven spread to lymph nodes or other sites (Figure 4-1). Cancers that are larger than 2 cm or involve regional lymph nodes are grouped into Stages II and III (Figures 4-2 - 4-4). Any cancer that has spread to another part of the body (e.g., lung, liver, bone) is Stage IV.

Doctors determine how aggressively to treat and manage an individual patient based on how advanced the cancer is locally in the breast and regionally in the lymph nodes. The greater the risk of microscopic cancer cell contamination throughout the body, MICROMETASTASIS, the greater the need for treatment to destroy these undetectable cancer cells. This treatment is called ADJUVANT THERAPY because it is most often administered after the surgery. Cancers proven upon initial evaluation to have spread to other organs (Stage IV, METASTATIC) represent the greatest management challenge. Treatment of such cancers is referred to as METASTATIC THERAPY.

| Stage 0 | Ti.s. | N0 | M0 |
|---|---|---|---|
| Stage I | T1 | N0 | M0 |
| Stage II A | T0, T1 | N1 | M0 |
| | T2 | N0 | M0 |
| Stage II B | T2 | N1 | M0 |
| | T3 | N0 | M0 |
| Stage III A | T0, T1, T2, | N2 | M0 |
| | T3 | N1, N2 | M0 |
| Stage III B | Any T | N3 | M0 |
| | T4 | Any N | M0 |
| Stage IV | Any T | Any N | M1 |

Table 4-1: TNM Staging System

Our evolving understanding of the biology of cancer necessitates continuous revisions to the staging criteria. Subcategories have been added to provide more definition like T1a,b,c and Stage IIa,b. Despite these ongoing revisions, a gap will always exist between scientific discovery and accepted policy. The clinical and pathologic findings, which fall outside of formal staging criteria but have an impact on patient outcome and the ability to predict risk of RECURRENCE or RELAPSE, are referred to as PROGNOSTIC CRITERIA.

The clinical and pathologic features that are the basis for prognostic criteria are further categorized as favorable or unfavorable. Prognostic features are generally less predictive of outcome than stage and do not always stand the test of time. Some tests like FLOW CYTOMETRY FOR S-PHASE and PLOIDY (ANEOPLOID, DIPLOID—measures of DNA instability) were once commonplace but are now less popular. Others like ESTROGEN RECEPTOR (ER) status and HER-2/NEU overexpression have become routine and are discussed later as we turn our attention to specific breast cancer treatments. The microscopic appearance of the cancer cells has also been used as a prognostic factor. This is referred to as NUCLEAR GRADE and HISTOLOGIC GRADE. A cancer cell that retains its ductal cell features is referred to as well differentiated and grade 1. A cancer cell that retains no defining features is referred to as undifferentiated and grade 4. Grade 2 is for moderately differentiated cells, and grade 3 refers to poorly differentiated cells. Like S-phase and ploidy, nuclear grade is also falling out of favor as more specific DNA markers like Her-2/neu replace it. Finally, some tests seem to be of recurring interest like Ki67, a nuclear protein present in dividing cells, an indicator of tumor proliferation that has been found to be a prognostic marker in breast cancer.

I explained to Jill and Greg that her tumor was small, 1.1 cm, or T1c, but the single contaminated sentinel node, N1a, resulted in her final stage of breast cancer being a Stage IIa. Additionally, the cancer was estrogen sensitive or ER+, which is considered favorable. The cancer cells were also tested in the pathology laboratory to see whether they had increased amounts of the gene Her-2/neu. This was done using a screening test called the HERCEPTEST, which was intermediately positive so a confirmatory test called FLUORESCENT IN SITU HYBRIDIZATION (FISH) was performed. This test confirmed that the cancer cells had excess Her-2/neu. The amplified amounts of Her-2 was kind of a mixed signal. In its entirety, the staging and prognostic criteria predicted that surgery alone offered a 70% chance of cure or a 30% chance that she would have a relapse of this cancer during the next 10 years. However, additional treatments after her surgery (adjuvant systemic therapy) could reduce the risk of a recurrence by more than half.

Jill and Greg were not comforted that the odds of cure were in Jill's corner. They wanted nothing less than a 100% guarantee of cure. I explained that this was not possible, but since we could reduce the risk of relapse by greater than 50% with adjuvant systemic therapy, her overall probability of cure would approach 90%. We sat down for a lengthy discussion of the systemic treatment of cancer.

NOTE: The tumor and lymph nodes represented in these illustrations are below the skin surface and may not be visible to the unaided eye.

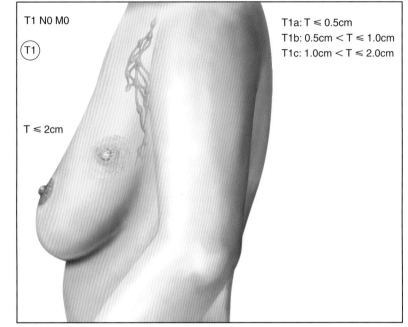

T1 N0 M0

(T1)

T ≤ 2cm

T1a: T ≤ 0.5cm
T1b: 0.5cm < T ≤ 1.0cm
T1c: 1.0cm < T ≤ 2.0cm

Figure 4-1: Stage I Disease

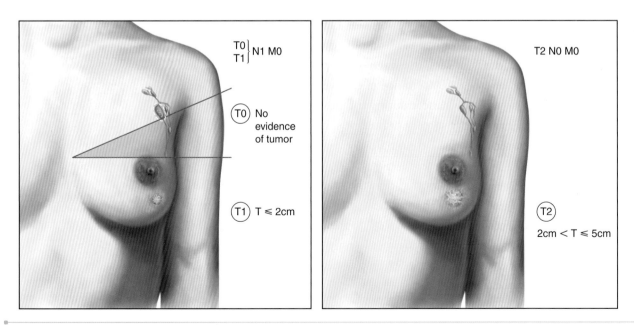

T0 }
T1 } N1 M0

(T0) No evidence of tumor

(T1) T ≤ 2cm

T2 N0 M0

(T2)

2cm < T ≤ 5cm

Figure 4-2: Stage II A Disease

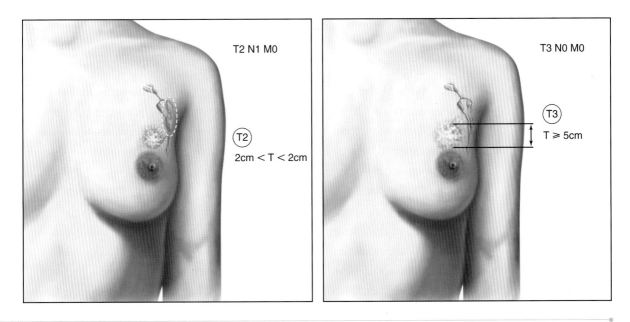

Figure 4-3: Stage II B Disease

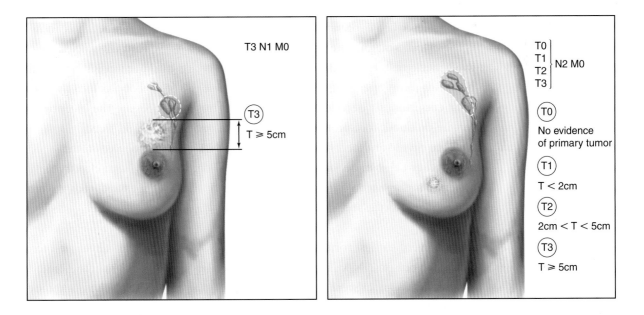

Figure 4-4: Stage III A Disease

# Systemic Therapy

The systemic theory of cancer argues that cancer is a cellular disease originating in an organ but possibly disseminated throughout the body at the time of diagnosis. If cancer cells are disseminated at the time of diagnosis, then loco-regional treatments are not adequate by themselves. Systemic or total body therapies are then needed to treat the entire body in order to destroy any undetectable microscopic contaminating disease (micrometastases) or proven cancer spread (metastases).

Efforts to seek and destroy the undetectable rogue cancer cells in the circulation, or the cancer cells nesting in proven metastatic deposits, have led to the development of an arsenal of weapons—medicines that travel in the blood, poisoning cancer cells wherever they nest. Jill asked how these medicines could cripple or destroy cancer cells. I answered by explaining how scientists examined cellular structure and function to find ways to disrupt the cancer cells' machinery.

To look at a cell in a scientific way, we would place it under a microscope. There we would see an outer cell membrane surrounding a gelatinous cytoplasm containing a nucleus at its core. Picture the Tootsie Pop, as described earlier, where the wrapper is the cell membrane, the candy is the cytoplasm, and the Tootsie Roll is the nucleus. Within the nucleus is the genetic material or DNA. The DNA is a coded information system like a blueprint or an operating code (the software of the cell). For a cell to live, it must continuously decode DNA messages. Those messages are the blueprint for the production of proteins, the cells' vital machinery. Additionally, for a cell to divide and become two cells, the DNA has to be copied so that the mother cell can divide into two identical daughter cells. An effective systemic therapy would need to interfere with the DNA messages that govern cell repair, growth, and division (Figure 4-5).

The very earliest forms of systemic therapy were chemicals developed to disrupt or poison DNA. The chemical agents first approved for the systemic treatment of cancer were called CHEMOTHERAPY. The logic of chemotherapy was straightforward: If cancer cells were dividing, they would have to copy their DNA to reproduce. If a treatment disrupted the DNA, the cells could

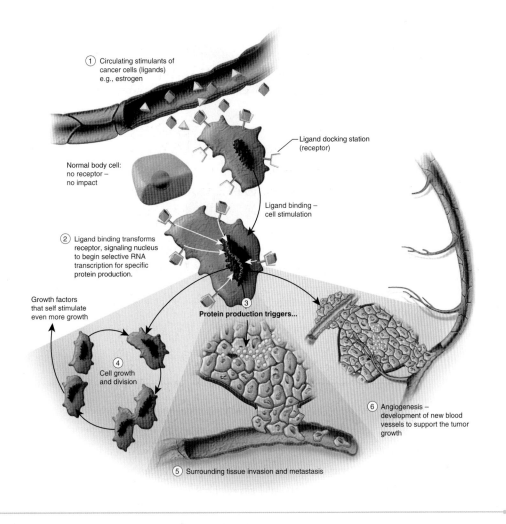

1 Circulating stimulants of cancer cells (ligands) e.g., estrogen

Ligand docking station (receptor)

Normal body cell: no receptor – no impact

Ligand binding – cell stimulation

2 Ligand binding transforms receptor, signaling nucleus to begin selective RNA transcription for specific protein production.

Growth factors that self stimulate even more growth

3 **Protein production triggers...**

4 Cell growth and division

6 Angiogenesis – development of new blood vessels to support the tumor growth

5 Surrounding tissue invasion and metastasis

Figure 4-5: Basic Model of Systemic Therapy (An effective treatment requires interference with the processes of cancer growth and proliferation.)

not divide and could not produce daughter cells. Without daughter cells, the cancer could not grow. Furthermore, if the DNA was disrupted, the messages for the production of proteins, the cell's vital machinery that allow the cell to eat, breathe, and remove waste, could not be uncoded. If the cell could not operate its intracellular machinery, the cancer cell would die. Thus, in theory, chemotherapy could stop the cancer growth and kill the cancer cells. Unfortunately, like cancer cells, all cells have DNA, and many cells in the body are also constantly growing and dividing: the hair cells, the blood cells, the cells that line the mouth and the intestinal tract, etc. Therefore, these DNA-disrupting drugs were also very toxic to normal cells (Figure 4-6).

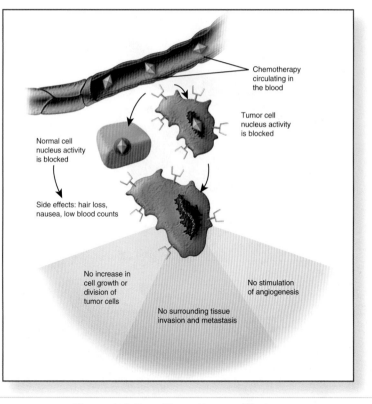

Figure 4-6: How Chemotherapy Works

Over the past three decades, great strides have been made to increase the effectiveness and decrease the toxicity of chemotherapy. Despite these improvements, both patients and physicians have demanded therapies that are safer, less toxic, and more cancer-cell specific. There was a call for "smart bombs" or "magic bullets" that could seek and destroy cancer cells without harm to the normal cell counterpart. These emerging new weapons in the arsenal against cancer have been called TARGETED THERAPY.

A cancer-specific treatment would by definition affect only cancer cells. However, these cancer cells are so genetically similar to normal cells that they escaped the recognition of the immune system. How could science accomplish what nature failed to do—target the cancer cells? The answer is in the DNA. In the past few decades, through ongoing work to translate the human genome (the basic DNA blueprint of all human cells), scientists are beginning to gain a deeper understanding of what makes a cancer cell behave the way it does. With these insights, cancer management is evolving. Cancer is no longer considered an organ disease or even a cellular one. Today, cancer is considered a genetic and molecular disease. Reflecting these changes, cancer therapy today is not just of a cellular nature, but also of a genetic and molecular nature.

Researchers now understand that within a given cell there are thousands of active genes (specific DNA codes) that define the cell's identity and function. These thousands of genes represent the codes for the thousands of proteins (molecules) that define the cell's structure and behavior. There may be only one tenth of 1% of those genes, one tenth of 1% of those important messages that go wrong or mutate, transforming a normal cell into a cancer cell. These mutations result in the overproduction or underproduction of critical proteins that control a cell's growth and behavior, causing that cell to become malignant or cancerous. If researchers could find the one tenth of 1% of those messages that are mutated, they could then target them specifically and create a magic bullet of cancer therapy. Doctors would then have a treatment that would be targeted only to the machinery gone awry in the cancer cell.

Targeted therapy may sound far-fetched, but history tells us otherwise. Antibiotics were the medical magic bullets of the last century, the targeted therapy of infectious diseases. For many centuries, infection was the leading cause of death in our society. Scientists began to develop treatments for infections by first understanding the molecular differences between bacterial cells and human cells. They were then able to target specific molecules unique to the bacteria, which in turn killed the bacteria and cured the infection without harming the cells of the human host.

As it turns out, targeted therapies for cancer have been around for some time. Observations of breast cancer remission after surgical removal of the ovaries were first reported over a century ago, revealing the relationship between ESTROGEN and breast cancer. Although sensitivity to estrogen is not unique to the mammary tissue of the breast, estrogen proved to be a powerful stimulant of some breast cancer cells. Antiestrogen therapy, like removing the ovaries surgically or taking antiestrogen pills, proved to be an effective weapon in the treatment of breast cancer while having minimal or modest effects on other normal cells of the body. This type of HORMONAL THERAPY, which has been in existence for over 40 years, was the first targeted molecular therapy. Today, hormonal therapies remain important components in the arsenal of treatments for breast and prostate cancers. HORMONES, like estrogen and testosterone can adhere to the surface of sensitive cells, like those of a breast or prostate cancer, triggering the DNA within the cancer cell to turn on and direct the manufacture of proteins that promote cell growth and division. The circulating hormone is referred to as a LIGAND and the structure that it adheres to on the cell membrane is referred to as a RECEPTOR. Interference with the ligand or receptor (e.g., an anti-estrogen pill) can down regulate the DNA of the cancer cell and in some cases cause cancer cell death.

Today we measure the breast cancer's sensitivity to estrogen by measuring a molecule called the ESTROGEN RECEPTOR on the cancer cell surface. The receptor is metaphorically a lock that estrogen (the key) can open and, in doing so, stimulate the cell to grow and divide. Understanding how estrogen stimulates the cancer cell has led to a rapidly expanding arsenal of hormonal therapies. These therapies that interfere with estrogen, by blocking its production or by preventing its interaction with the estrogen receptor on the cancer cell, prevent estrogen's stimulatory effects and cause sensitive cancers to go into remission. (Sensitivity to another sex hormone, PROGESTERONE, is also commonly measured; however, its predictive value is significantly less than estrogen, and, therefore, it is not discussed further.)

Although this sounds so straightforward, a lot of confusion exists surrounding hormonal treatment of breast cancer, primarily because of the medical establishment's failure to speak a consistent language. Women who have been diagnosed with breast cancer are told that they cannot have or must stop hormone replacement therapy, then in the same breath they are prescribed "hormonal therapy" to treat the cancer. The patient is told that she is menopausal and that she is not making estrogen, and then she is prescribed an antiestrogen therapy to block the estrogen that she was just told she is not making. Why is she given hormonal

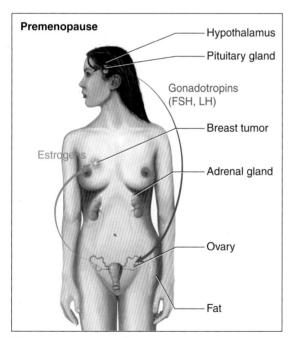

Premenopause

— Hypothalamus
— Pituitary gland

Gonadotropins
(FSH, LH)

— Breast tumor

Estrogens

— Adrenal gland

— Ovary

— Fat

Woman: premenopausal, estrogen produced by ovary

Figure 4-7: Estrogen Receptor–Premenopausal

therapy when she cannot have hormones? Why is she given an antiestrogen therapy if she does not make estrogen?

Hormones are chemical messengers that are made in one part of the body and travel through the blood to other parts of the body where they have some effect. In the blood, there may be as many as a hundred distinct hormones that affect everything from menstruation, lactation, and pregnancy to metabolism and chemical balance. The hormones are categorized into groups, one of which is the sex hormones. Sex hormones are made in the ovary, testicle, and adrenal gland. Estrogen, made in the ovary, is the sex hormone that we associate with women, as its production at puberty stimulates the development of female secondary sexual characteristics; its decline in middle age signals menopause. Because the

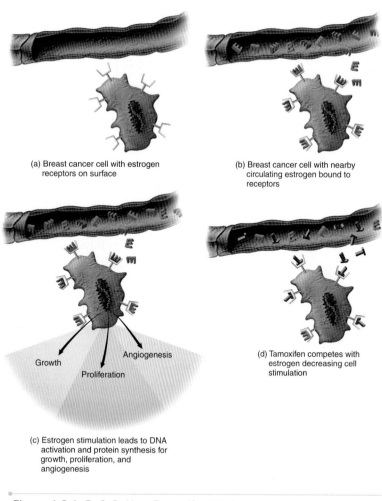

(a) Breast cancer cell with estrogen receptors on surface

(b) Breast cancer cell with nearby circulating estrogen bound to receptors

Growth    Angiogenesis
    Proliferation

(c) Estrogen stimulation leads to DNA activation and protein synthesis for growth, proliferation, and angiogenesis

(d) Tamoxifen competes with estrogen decreasing cell stimulation

Figure 4-8 A, B, C, D: How Tamoxifen Works

mammary tissue of the breast develops under the influence of estrogen, it is not surprising that many mammary cancers often retain estrogen sensitivity. Such an estrogen-sensitive cancer cell is stimulated to grow and divide when circulating estrogen binds to the estrogen receptors on the cell's surface (Figure 4-8).

Understanding the physiology of estrogen production was critical to the design of interference strategies that could prevent circulating estrogen from stimulating cancer cells in at-risk women. Possible interference mechanisms include: Preventing stimulation of the ovaries by lutenizing hormone-release hormone (LHRH) released by the pituitary gland, thereby stopping ovarian production of estrogen (treatment = LHRH Agonist). Removing the ovaries (treatment = SURGICAL OOPHERECTOMY). Blocking estrogen receptors on cancer cells from binding with estrogen (treatment = TAMOXIFEN). Destroying the estrogen receptor on the cancer cell surface (treatment = SERM). And interfering with any non-ovarian estrogen production (treatment = AROMATASE INHIBITOR). A more detailed discussion is in order.

In a premenopausal woman, stopping estrogen stimulation requires removing the source of estrogen, the ovary, or blocking the estrogen receptor to prevent estrogen binding. Estrogen receptors are present on many kinds of cells, not just mammary, which is why menopause has so many consequences. Scientists have tried to design drugs that will selectively block only the receptors on mammary cells. These drugs are called SELECTIVE ESTROGEN RECEPTOR MODULATORS (SERM), and two have been approved by the Food and Drug Administration: TAMOXIFEN (Nolvadex) and RALOXIFENE (Evista). Tamoxifen is the only SERM approved to treat invasive breast cancer. And it is the only anti-estrogen therapy currently approved for invasive breast cancer in premenopausal women (those who still have regular menses). Additionally only tamoxifen has been approved as a breast cancer prevention drug in pre-menopausal women. As of this writing, Raloxifene use is limited to breast cancer prevention in post-menopausal women. Unfortunately, neither drug is perfectly selective, and thus, they still cause some unwanted SIDE EFFECTS.

As a woman approaches her fifth or sixth decade of life, the ovaries stop producing estrogen, which results in menopause and the symptoms referred to as "change of life." In truth, estrogen levels fall very low but not to zero. Although ovarian estrogen output may cease, an adrenal sex hormone is transformed into estrogen by an ENZYME, (called AROMATASE) found primarily in fat cells. Thus, even after menopause a woman still has some circulating estrogen. Stopping estrogen stimulation of mammary cancer cells in a post-menopausal woman thus requires either blocking the receptor with a SERM or disrupting the aromatase enzyme so that it cannot convert the adrenal hormone into estrogen. The class of drugs developed to block the aromatase reaction is called AROMATASE INHIBITORS (Figure 4-9).

SERMs competitively inhibit the binding of estrogen to the estrogen receptor. Oopherectomy removes the ovaries that produce estrogen in menstruating

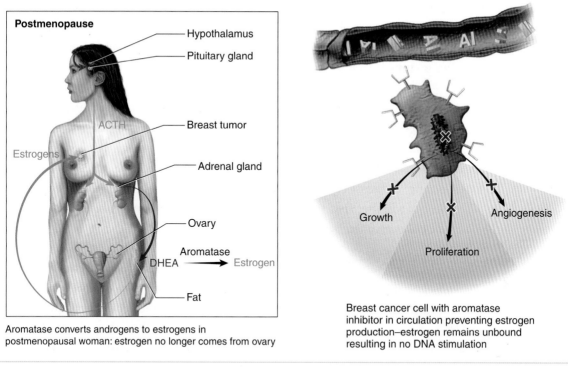

**Postmenopause**

- Hypothalamus
- Pituitary gland
- Breast tumor
- Adrenal gland
- Ovary

ACTH

Estrogens

Aromatase
DHEA → Estrogen

- Fat

Growth

Proliferation

Angiogenesis

Aromatase converts androgens to estrogens in postmenopausal woman: estrogen no longer comes from ovary

Breast cancer cell with aromatase inhibitor in circulation preventing estrogen production—estrogen remains unbound resulting in no DNA stimulation

Figure 4-9: Estrogen Receptor–Postmenopausal        Figure 4-9 A: How Aromatase Inhibitors Work

women. And aromatase inhibitors prevent estrogen production in post meno-pausal women. FASLODEX (FULVESTRANT), however, works directly to destroy the estrogen receptor. Studies comparing it to aromatase inhibitors found it equally effective. It is currently approved for the treatment of advanced estrogen receptor positive (ER+) invasive breast cancer in post-menopausal women and is being actively investigated in pre-menopausal women.

Lastly, the idea of shutting down ovarian estrogen production without the perceived drastic measure of surgical removal of the ovaries has piqued the interest of researchers for some time. Such a treatment has also been of keen interest for those women who, despite taking tamoxifen, continue to menstruate, suggesting inadequate estrogen receptor blockade. (Most women on tamoxifen stop menstruating as estrogen receptors are blocked on all sensitive tissues, including the uterus.) A class of drug that can achieve reversible medical castration of the ovaries is the lutenizing hormone-release hormone (LHRH) agonist. When injected this drug fools the ovary by creating a biochemical/hormonal environment similar to the part of the menstrual cycle in which estrogen is not produced. Although not yet approved by the FDA for breast cancer it is approved in genecologic diseases that require reversible cessation of menses and is being actively researched as a breast cancer treatment.

Our improved understanding allows us to develop a clear and consistent language about hormones and breast cancer. The expression "estrogen replacement therapy" should replace "hormone replacement therapy." The expression "antiestrogen treatment" of breast cancer should replace "hormonal therapy" of breast cancer. Antiestrogen therapy should be further specified to identify whether that therapy is a SERM, an aromatase inhibitor, Faslodex, or an LHRH agonist.

**Many breast cancer patients are advised never to take hormones because hormones could activate the cancer. In reality, they should avoid estrogen, just one of the sex hormones in the body.**

Although doctors have known about the estrogen relationship for a century and have been able to test cancer cells routinely for the estrogen receptor for over two decades, other molecular targets have been much more difficult to define. Today, over 400 molecular and genetic targets and their respective interference therapies are being investigated. The targets include receptors on the cell surface, the ligands that bind to them, the DNA which is stimulated by the transformed receptor, the RNA translation of the DNA, the proteins which the RNA define, etc. (Figure 4-10)

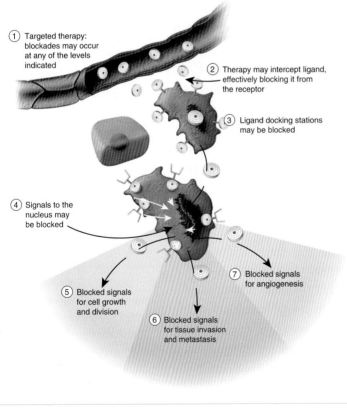

① Targeted therapy: blockades may occur at any of the levels indicated

② Therapy may intercept ligand, effectively blocking it from the receptor

③ Ligand docking stations may be blocked

④ Signals to the nucleus may be blocked

⑤ Blocked signals for cell growth and division

⑥ Blocked signals for tissue invasion and metastasis

⑦ Blocked signals for angiogenesis

Figure 4-10: How Target Therapy Works

Thus far, two targets, HER-2/NEU and VEGF have resulted in targeted therapies that have been approved for breast cancer. Scientists became interested in Her-2/neu (Her-2) due to observations that, when activated in breast cancer cells, which happens to be about 25% of the time, those cell have behaved more aggressively. Two drugs have been developed to target the protein encoded by the Her-2/neu gene, HERCEPTIN and TYKERB. Herceptin has been proven to shrink metastases from some breast cancers that have excess or amplified amounts of Her-2 gene as well as prevent recurrences of the Her-2 amplified cancers when administered as part of adjuvant therapy. The other Her-2 targeted therapy, Tykerb, interferes with the Her-2 receptor but differently than Herceptin. Tykerb has thus far only been approved for the treatment of metastatic cancer. AVASTIN (BEVACIZUMAB) interferes with a different target, VEGF (VASCULAR ENDOTHELIAL GROWTH FACTOR). Both Tykerb and Avastin have been more recently approved by the FDA than Herceptin, thus they have more limited indications. The clinical trials leading to the approval of theses targeted therapies tested the hypothesis that the standard of care (chemotherapy) plus an experimental therapy (targeted) is superior to standard therapy (chemo) alone. Thus most targeted therapies are administered with chemo. Ongoing research is evaluating targeted therapies in combination with each other without concurrent chemotherapy.

Today, not only do doctors need to understand the tumor characteristics, the node status, and whether there is any evidence of spread to other organs of the body, but they also need to know the cancer's sensitivity to estrogen and the extent to which the cancer overproduces Her-2. All of these features have an impact on the local, regional, and systemic therapies that are recommended.

Jill and Greg were a bit overwhelmed. Her cancer was small but node positive, ER+ and Her-2 positive as well. These findings seem conflicting; small tumor and ER+ were favorable, whereas node positive and Her-2 positive were less favorable. Would Jill be required to take chemotherapy alone, chemotherapy with Herceptin, or chemotherapy with Herceptin and an anti-estrogen? I suggested a deep breath and counting to 10 as I took a moment to summarize what we had discussed so far. First, our understanding of cancer has evolved from the disease of an organ to a systemic cellular disease to a genetic and molecular disease. Second, there is a need for adjuvant systemic therapies in patients who are at risk for microscopic systemic contamination. Third, the staging system in conjunction with prognostic factors allows us to predict the risk of microscopic systemic contamination. Fourth, systemic therapies are of three types: chemotherapy, antiestrogen treatment, and the newest type of treatment, targeted therapy. Now we needed to discuss how oncologists select and integrate these treatments for each patient.

# Current Treatment of Breast Cancer

Jill and Greg remained anxious as I began to explain the treatment for a Stage IIa breast cancer with an involved lymph node that was both estrogen receptor positive and Her-2 amplified. I said that there may be treatment options. Some of the possible treatments are considered standard, whereas others would require participation in a CLINICAL TRIAL. Their eyes started to glaze over. Jill and Greg may have been feeling overwhelmed, but I was undeterred as my responsibility was to provide all the information needed for them to make an informed decision about Jill's treatment. An informed decision required knowledge of both standard therapy and the clinical trials for which she was eligible. I decided some background on how a standard treatment is established and what a clinical trial is might provide a better context in which to understand the treatment options.

For any systemic treatment to become a standard of care it must complete a long and complicated evaluation. The evaluation process incorporates three specific phases of testing. The treatment must first be proven safe (PHASE 1), then effective (PHASE 2), and then better than the current standard of care that it is replacing (PHASE 3). Remarkably, this process can take up to 12 years. Just as the surgical approach to the management of locoregional disease progressed over the past 30 years from the radical mastectomy to the lumpectomy with sentinel lymph node biopsy, so too has the systemic management of breast cancer evolved. This evolution occurred on two related fronts: the development of effective treatments for proven metastases and the use of those active treatments in the adjuvant setting. Effective metastatic treatments are those that reduce symptoms and prolong the life of patients with advanced cancer. Effective adjuvant treatments are those that reduce the relative risk of cancer recurrence or more simply increase the chance of cure.

The beginning of this scientific evolution can be found in the laboratory research of the late 1940s, which confirmed that certain chemicals could kill cancer cells. A decade later, the first chemotherapy drugs were administered to patients with metastatic cancer. By 1968, the chemotherapy treatment of patients with metastatic breast cancer was becoming routine. More importantly, the first reports of surgical adjuvant chemotherapy were published. Breast surgeons united to advance the science of breast cancer treatment, leading to the formation of one of the largest and most successful cooperative research organizations, the NATIONAL SURGICAL ADJUVANT BREAST AND BOWEL PROJECT (NSABP). Another decade passed before researchers could confirm that polychemotherapy (also called multidrug or combination chemotherapy) offered superior results to single-drug treatment. The first internationally recognized combination therapy was titled CMF, an acronym for the three drugs: Cytoxan, Methotrexate, and Fluorouracil.

The 1980s brought the introduction of a new class of chemotherapy drugs related to antibiotics, the ANTHRACYCLINES. The anthracycline antibiotic, DOXORUBICIN (ADRIAMYCIN), proved to be the most active drug to date in breast cancer therapy. Combination chemotherapy with Adriamycin (CAF/FAC) replaced CMF in metastatic disease and was increasingly used in higher risk node-positive patients. Attempts to evaluate the impact of modifications of drug doses and drug delivery schedules confirmed that six months of therapy were as effective as 12 months, but diluting the therapy by giving lower or less frequent doses compromised effectiveness. These studies helped to establish optimal dose and schedule, maximizing chemotherapy benefit and limiting toxicity.

The 1990s had successes and failures. A new class of chemotherapy drugs was introduced, TAXANES, with activity comparable to Adriamycin. Today, three taxane drugs are approved for the treatment of patients with breast cancer, PACLITAXEL (TAXOL), DOCETAXEL (TAXOTERE) and NAB-PACLITAXEL (ABRAXANE). Antiestrogen therapy was advanced with the approval of aromatase inhibitors. Theses agents were invaluable additions to the arsenal of weapons. The benefit of chemotherapy was confirmed in node-negative disease, and the additive benefit of chemotherapy plus antiestrogen therapy was proven. A new category of treatments, SUPPORT DRUGS, was introduced. These drugs have significantly improved the QUALITY OF LIFE of the cancer patient. Unfortunately, there were also disappointments. Dose-intensive regimens supported by BONE

MARROW stem cells, often referred to as bone marrow transplant, did not lead to highly anticipated increased cure rates. The close of the decade brought the first targeted molecular therapy, Herceptin, from the research bench to the treatment clinic.

The decade and for that matter the century and millennium beginning with the year 2000 will be memorable in cancer medicine. Since the 1960s, cancer researchers believed that paradigm-changing cancer treatment strategies could only happen with an improved understanding of the genetic and thereby molecular basis of cancer. They were so right. I believe the birth of the third millennium will be regarded as the sea change in the history of cancer treatment. Forty years of bench research finally revolutionized the way cancer patients are screened, diagnosed, treated and supported. Understanding the genetic basis of cancer led to the development of a new class of systemic treatments, targeted therapies, with three drugs approved as of this writing and more than 400 in development. The first of these to be approved, Herceptin, has had such a dramatic impact on cure that the entire approach to the patient with invasive cancer has changed. Today, sensitivity to Herceptin is the pivotal decision point in treatment planning, more important than tumor size and node status.

Despite all attempts at the intelligent design of new therapeutics, not every exciting drug prospect succeeds in clinical testing while others have unexpected benefits. Among the surprises is a class of drugs developed to improve bone health in women, the BISPHOSPHONATES. They were originally developed as a treatment to prevent the leaching of calcium from bone in patients with metastatic cancer in the bone. They were subsequently proven beneficial in slowing the bone loss of OSTEOPOROSIS. Their proven benefit in preserving bone health suggested a role in the prevention of accelerated bone loss often observed in breast cancer patients on antiestrogen therapies. Trials were designed and initiated in which breast cancer patients on antiestrogen treatments were randomized to also receive a bisphosphonate. Investigators were surprised to find that the addition of the bisphosphonate appeared to improve the cure rate by preventing cancer relapses, and not only bone recurrences. Confirmatory trials are underway but the fact that two different trials have reached similar conclusions have made Bisphosphonates and the role of bone physiology in cancer two of the hottest topics in cancer research.

Today, an ever-increasing volume of medical research has resulted in some very provocative Phase II (evaluating the effectiveness of treatment) results. Unfortunately, Phase II clinical trial results leave many unanswered questions for the patients of this new millennium: How and when should they incorporate new drugs in adjuvant treatment? What is the role of the emerging arsenal of targeted therapies in the management of breast cancer, and how and when should they be incorporated? Should systemic therapy be introduced after biopsy, but before definitive surgery (termed NEOADJUVANT or PRIMARY SYSTEMIC therapy)? Results from Phase II testing, regardless of the enthusiasm with which they are reported and received, still require Phase III testing for conclusive proof of superiority. Only then do they warrant a change in the standard of care. Unfortunately, Phase III testing of adjuvant treatments may take five to seven years to complete, leaving the physician and the patient to grapple with unproven options as treatment is planned.

I presented Jill and Greg with a nationally conducted, clinical trial. I thought that this study represented her best option, as it not only offered her standard-of-care chemotherapy with Herceptin and five years of antiestrogen treatment, but also, it offered the possibility of Jill receiving an additional therapy.

Jill and Greg had to share in this important decision about participating in a clinical trial. Before Jill could be enrolled, they would need to sign an informed consent document, attesting to their complete understanding of all risks and benefits associated with the treatment. This was the beginning of the second most difficult job I have as a medical oncologist, explaining and comparing the risks and benefits of a clinical trial with standard treatment.

## The Language of Clinical Outcomes

Explaining treatment risks and benefits can be complicated in the best of situations. Unfortunately, because the medical establishment has not standardized the language of treatment-related measures and outcomes, this process can be a nightmare. The language of the oncologist can be very confusing. Even the word "cancer" is not uniformly used but may be substituted by malignant growth, cancerous tumor, NEOPLASM, etc. The outcomes of treatment are even more confusing for patients to understand as terms such as REMISSION, RESPONSE, RECURRENCE, PROGRESSION, and SURVIVAL are used to express the outcomes of therapy. Worse, for each of these outcomes, such as remission or response, a myriad of qualifiers will be added, including minor, partial, complete, clinical, radiographic, and pathologic. The terms progression and survival may be used in conjunction with or as an alternative to remission and response and then further refined or more likely confused by qualifying descriptive phrases such as FREEDOM FROM PROGRESSION, RELAPSE-FREE PROGRESSION, TIME TO PROGRESSION, OVERALL SURVIVAL, and DISEASE-SPECIFIC SURVIVAL. If this was not confusing enough, these outcome measurements are reported as statistical probabilities, which are usually relative rather than absolute. It often sounds like double talk. How can patients and their loved ones be expected to understand? They just want to know if they will be cured.

Unbelievably, it gets worse. Many different clinical trials are conducted on each specific treatment to evaluate its effectiveness and to generate outcomes, but because the trial designs are not identical, the results are not either. The oncologist not only has to present this confusing data with confusing words but also he or she may have to present it for two or three trials, none of which used the same outcomes or reached the same conclusions.

In this era of patient empowerment and shared decision making, after the dizzying display of data, the doctor is supposed to ask the patient what he or she wants to do. The thoroughly confused patient often responds, "What would you recommend to your wife or mother?"

It does not have to be this way, and it should not. It is clear to me after more than 20 years of caring for cancer patients that there needs to be a consensus among oncologists on how data are reported and presented to patients so that the words are meaningful, the discussed risks and benefits are absolute, and the data can be compared. A researcher, Peter Ravdin, has published such an approach, and it has been made available to patients and physicians through an Internet site: *www.adjuvantonline.com*. I have begun using this simple method, which poses the question: "What would happen to 100 patients such as yourself if…" The approach is straightforward and can be quite illuminating, as my discussion with Greg and Jill illustrates. The questions Jill, Greg, and I posed were as follows: What would happen to 100 women like Jill if she did no further treatment? What would happen to 100 women like Jill if she took an antiestrogen pill only? What would happen to 100 women like Jill if she took only chemotherapy? What would happen to 100 women like Jill if she underwent chemotherapy with a sequential anthracycline plus taxane regimen with Herceptin and in addition she underwent five years of anti-estrogen treatment with tamoxifen?

Answers to these questions are made possible by a computer analysis, which creates an age- and risk factor-adjusted assessment of cancer cure based on a huge dataset, including all relevant Phase III clinical trials. This type of data comparison, where many related but not identical clinical trials are combined, is called a META-ANALYSIS and is very valuable in assessing risk for large patient populations. The dataset is further updated on a continuous basis so that the most recently completed Phase III trials can be included in the assessment.

The analysis begins by sitting together at the computer and entering the necessary data. The online program requests information about the patient and final pathology. Jill and Greg huddled close as I typed in her age, TNM staging, and estrogen sensitivity. All that was left was to hit enter, and then the computer analysis would be under way.

The first question posed was this: Over the next 10 years, what would happen to 100 women like Jill if they chose no adjuvant systemic treatment? Studies suggest 69 women would be cured by the surgery, free of cancer. Thirty of the remaining 31 women would relapse with breast cancer metastases. One woman would die of a cause unrelated to the breast cancer. Most unfortunately, the majority of those who relapse would eventually die from the breast cancer.

The second question posed in the computer analysis was this: Over the next 10 years, what would happen to 100 women like Jill if they chose adjuvant antiestrogen therapy? Studies suggest that seven fewer women would relapse. Seventy-six women would be alive, well and free of cancer; however, 23 would have relapsed, likely to die of cancer.

The third question posed in the computer survey was this: What would happen to 100 women like Jill if adjuvant chemotherapy with a sequential anthracycline plus taxane was used? Studies suggest that the chemotherapy would save the lives of 10 women. Seventy-nine women would be alive and well, free of cancer relapse, whereas 20 women would succumb to the cancer.

The final question posed was this: Over the next 10 years, what would happen to 100 women like Jill if they chose the adjuvant chemotherapy in addition to antiestrogen therapy? The combined therapy would cure 15 more women not cured by the surgery. Eighty-four would remain alive, well and free of cancer. Only 15 women would relapse and risk cancer death. Once again one woman would die of an unrelated cause (Figure 4-11).

Unfortunately, we could not obtain the answer to the query that is of the greatest interest: What would happen to 100 women like Jill if chemotherapy was administered with Herceptin and followed by five years of antiestrogen therapy? Just like the research, it relies upon Adjuvant Online continues to evolve. As of this writing—the 9th update which will include the data set on adjuvant Herceptin benefit—is still in development. So I explained to Jill and Greg that the pivotal Phase III trial leading to Herceptin's approval in adjuvant therapy decreased the five-year relapse rate by 50% compared to chemotherapy alone. If that trial data holds up at 10 years, then our model would show 90 women alive and free of cancer and only ten relapsed.

Figure 4-11: Adjuvantonline: Shared Decision Making

An oncologist might review this information on surgery, chemotherapy, Herceptin, and antiestrogen treatments and report that the overall cure rate is 90%, but that would not explain the specific contribution of each component of therapy. Restricting our discussion to Figure 4–11, we might say the cure rate of adjuvant combined chemo/antiestrogen therapy is 50% because 15 of 30 women who were destined to relapse were cured. Another way this is reported is a 50% reduction in the "relative" risk of recurrence and death. It may be a more appropriate measure to say that the cure rate of chemotherapy and antiestrogen treatment is 15%, as 15 women of the 100 are cured specifically because of the combined adjuvant therapy. In other words, there is a reduction in the "absolute" risk of recurrence and death of 15%. Eight women of the 100 are cured specifically because of the contribution of chemotherapy. Is that 8% absolute improvement in cure worth the additional cost and suffering associated with the treatment? What if that benefit was only 3%? Each patient must answer that question but only with data that are clearly presented and meaningful.

When the data are presented in this way, it becomes clear that only 15 of the 100 women will truly benefit from the treatment, yet all 100 will be treated. As I explained to Jill and Greg, science has yet to develop technology that can detect micrometastases. There is no way to know who are the 69 women already cured by the surgery or who are the 15 women destined to relapse despite taking chemotherapy and antiestrogen treatment. Thus, all 100 women are treated: 69 who have no need because they are cured by surgery, 15 who have no need because it will not help, and 15 who will be truly cured by this intervention.

Jill and Greg found the discussion encouraging. Undergoing outpatient chemotherapy for four months, Herceptin for one year, followed by five years of tamoxifen seemed a small cost to cut in half her risk of relapse. Jill became excited when she had a sudden realization that the analysis did not include the additional therapy being studied in the clinical trial, which might further increase her chance of cure. The reason that the additional therapy was not included in the analysis is that Phase III studies evaluating its role in the adjuvant setting have not been concluded. This means that we do not currently know whether this additional therapy may benefit patients like Jill, and more importantly, we do not know what toxicities the addition may cause.

It seemed like a good time to review what we had discussed so far. The systemic therapy of cancer has evolved by demonstrating a treatment's ability to reduce the size of the cancer, prolong life, and improve its quality. Sequential improvements in therapy have been accomplished using a standardized three-phase approach, which confirms safety (Phase I), efficacy (Phase II), and superiority (Phase III). The process is continuous such that at any moment hundreds of research studies are ongoing in each phase. Studies not only evaluate new systemic therapies, alone and in combination, but also evaluate how to best integrate these therapies with the locoregional modalities of surgery and radiation. This dynamic and constantly improving treatment landscape may be exciting for researchers and may provide encouragement for those at risk like Jill, but it can also pose a dilemma for the patient and doctor who want to use all of the resources available to maximize the opportunity for cure and survival. Patients such as Jill and Greg, their loved ones, as well as their doctors often need some direction, some authority to pronounce a current standard of care, define reasonable alternatives when a standard does not exist, and provide guidance for patients who wish to pursue a clinical trial option. This was my next topic of discussion with Jill and Greg.

## The Standard of Care

Nationally and internationally, oncologists and cancer researchers have recognized the problems that the abundance of emerging data creates for making a treatment decision. The oncology community has responded by creating a system for peer review, discussion, and dissemination of new research. Data are released at designated meetings and in professional journals.

The oncology community has also responded by developing cooperative clinical research groups, such as the National Surgical Adjuvant Breast and Bowel Project, to provide broad patient access to new therapies in Phase II and Phase III testing. Consensus conferences, developed by the National Comprehensive Cancer Center Network, the American Society of Clinical Oncology, and the National Cancer Institute, have been organized to review emerging data and to provide a consensus on patient management.

The following discussions reflect those most recent consensus statements on stage-specific therapies and when and how to integrate new therapeutics into clinical practice.

## DCIS

The treatment of DCIS has evolved substantially over the past decade, with the majority of women now being treated with breast-conserving surgery. The DCIS guidelines use size and extent of the breast tumor, grade, and margin status in identifying appropriate treatment.

Women with small (< 5 mm), low-grade, pure DCIS can be offered excision to negative margins followed by observation. This appropriate therapy is an alternative to radiation or simple mastectomy. For women with a DCIS lesion of greater than 5 mm that is not widespread, the available evidence from randomized trials demonstrates that radiation after excision to negative pathologic margins is effective. Simple mastectomy without intentional axillary lymph node removal is also considered an appropriate option. Women with widespread DCIS or with documented involvement of two or more quadrants of the breast should be treated with only simple mastectomy. Regardless of the local breast treatment, if the tumor is ER+, five years of antiestrogen therapy is recommended to decrease risk of future breast cancer. Currently only tamoxifen is approved for this indication.

## Locoregional Therapy and Stage I and Stage II Invasive Breast-Cancer

Numerous trials have consistently demonstrated that modified radical mastectomy and breast conservation surgery (complete tumor excision, axillary lymph node evaluation, and breast irradiation) are equally effective at making patients disease free and both result in equally good survival rates. A number of factors influence the choice between the local therapies, including relative contraindications to breast conservation surgery (extensive DCIS, nipple/areolar involvement, large tumor, poor cosmesis), patient preference, and available medical expertise and facilities. Other factors, such as the potential for inherited susceptibility, may also be important to consider when determining the course of therapy.

The risk of chest wall recurrence is high enough in women with primary invasive cancers greater than 5 cm or with four or more involved axillary lymph nodes the use of postmastectomy locoregional irradiation in order to decrease the MORBIDITY of locoregional recurrence. Substantial controversy exists regarding the use of chest wall and regional lymph node irradiation in women with lesions less than 5 cm and with one to three involved axillary lymph nodes. An ongoing clinical trial—in which women with one to three positive lymph nodes postmastectomy are randomized to radiation versus no radiation—will hopefully resolve this issue.

## Adjuvant Systemic Therapy for Stages I, II, and IIIa Invasive Breast Cancer

Our expanded understanding of the genetic and molecular underpinning of breast cancer has truly changed the paradigm of adjuvant systemic therapy. Estrogen receptor status and Her-2/neu status have eclipsed in importance tumor size and axillary lymph node status in regard to the selection of adjuvant systemic therapy.

Testing of estrogen and progesterone receptor status as well as Her-2/neu status should be done on all newly diagnosed primary invasive breast cancers. Patients with invasive breast cancers that are estrogen and/or progesterone receptor positive should be considered for adjuvant antiestrogen therapy. Adjuvant antiestrogen therapy is recommended for women with estrogen receptor-positive breast cancer regardless of menopausal status, age, or Her-2/neu status.

Tumor-specific genetic profiling, currently available through the ONCO-TYPE DX test, should be considered in all ER+, node negative, Her-2 negative tumors larger than 0.5 cm in order to assess the role of concomitant chemotherapy. Oncotype DX is a special pathology test that analyzes the expression of certain genes in a breast cancer. It can help predict a patient's breast cancer-related prognosis and the potential benefit of chemotherapy in addition to antiestrogen treatment. Oncotype DX results are not used to make a decision about who should receive antiestrogen therapy, as all ER+ patients should have five years of antiestrogen treatment. Other gene profiling tests are in development. One, branded MAMMO PRINT, was recently approved by the FDA.

Primary invasive breast cancers larger than 0.5 cm that over-express the HER-2/neu gene as determined by a three-plus Herceptest (+++) or by gene amplification documented by FISH testing (>2.4 copies/cell) should receive adjuvant Herceptin. As of this writing adjuvant Herceptin should be given initially with chemotherapy then continued to complete one year of therapy.

All consensus guidelines continue to recommend the use of adjuvant polychemotherapy (multidrugs or combination chemotherapy) in the treatment of women with invasive breast cancer whose tumors neither stain positive for the estrogen receptor (ER–) nor demonstrate amplified Her-2/neu (Her2-). The guidelines recommend the use of polychemotherapy in all women under 70 years of age with lymph node-positive breast cancer, as well as women with node negative tumors greater than 1.0 cm. Guidelines recommend consideration of polychemotherapy for women with ER–, lymph node-negative breast cancer 0.6 cm to 1.0 cm in greatest diameter if any unfavorable features are present (e.g., angiolymphatic invasion, high S-phase, high nuclear grade, high histologic grade).

## Selection of Optimal Adjuvant Systemic Therapy

All patients with estrogen receptor-positive tumors should receive antiestrogen treatment for five years. Premenopausal patients should be offered oophorectomy or tamoxifen. Postmenopausal patients should receive treatment with an aromatase inhibitor. The improved outcomes achieved with aromatase inhibitors over tamoxifen in post-menopausal women suggest that those women already receiving tamoxifen in the adjuvant setting who become menopausal during treatment should consider either changing to an aromatase inhibitor or sequentially taking an aromatase inhibitor for at least two years after completion of their five-year tamoxifen therapy. Even if other systemic therapy (chemotherapy, Her-2 based) is recommended, five years of antiestrogen therapy is the current standard of care in all estrogen receptor- and progesterone receptor-postive patients. Patients with estrogen receptor-negative tumors should not be offered adjuvant therapy with an antiestrogen.

The treatment of choice for patients with estrogen receptor-negative, Her-2 negative tumors is combination chemotherapy. Low-risk patients, those with small tumors (T1), no lymph node involvement (N0), and favorable prognostic factors may be adequately treated with the chemotherapy doublet of Taxotere plus Cytoxan. Patients with larger tumors (T2, T3) or node positive disease are recommended to receive adjuvant chemotherapy containing both a taxane and an anthracycline either in combination or in sequence.

Her-2 positive tumors greater than 5 mm (regardless of ER status and node status) should receive one year of adjuvant Herceptin if not enrolled in a clinical trial. As all Herceptin adjuvant trials start the one year of Herceptin treatment in conjunction with chemotherapy, only such an approach can be recommended. Anthracyclines should not be administered with Herseptin, due to cardiac risks.

Optimally performed interventions provide the greatest benefits. Chemotherapy is no substitute for good surgery or vice versa. The combined use of optimal surgery, chemotherapy, Herceptin, antiestrogen therapy, and radiotherapy has a major impact on the risk of recurrence.

Jill and Greg found the discussion about informed consent a bit overwhelming. They decided that their best treatment option was a combination chemotherapy program in which a four-cycle course of Adriamycin and Cytoxan would be followed in sequence by a course of a taxane with Herceptin. Based on our discussions and their own research, this combination offered the best reduction in recurrence risk that could be achieved with chemotherapy. After chemotherapy, antiestrogen therapy consisting of a five-year course of a daily antiestrogen pill (tamoxifen, because Jill is premenopausal) would further reduce the risk of a relapse.

Jill and Greg were concerned that this plan did not include some of the new treatments they had read about on the Internet. I explained that these emerging targeted therapies are relatively new. Phase III testing of new therapeutics must first be performed. Although some of these drug therapies proved effective in Phase III testing in metastatic patients, leading to their approval by the Food and Drug Administration and their place in the arsenal of systemic therapies used in the care of patients with metastatic disease, Phase III testing in the adjuvant setting would need to be successfully completed before they could be used for patients with more limited cancer like Jill. The clinical trial that Jill and Greg had reviewed was addressing the very question of whether adding an additional therapy to a standard chemotherapy plus Herceptin, and an antiestrogen therapy in women with ER+, Her-2 positive, node-positive breast cancer might further reduce the risk of recurrence without unacceptable toxicity.

# Shared Decision Making

After a bit more deliberation, participating in the clinical trial seemed like a reasonable solution to all of Jill's concerns, but Greg seemed hesitant. He was concerned that she might enroll in the trial but not receive the additional therapy. Greg was correct. In order to prove that a therapeutic drug adds benefit, clinical trials are structured so that some of the patients receive the current standard of care, whereas others receive the standard treatment plus the additional therapy under investigation. This kind of trial design is the most common and is referred to as RANDOMIZED, where patients are randomly assigned to receive either the standard treatment or the standard treatment plus the additional therapy being evaluated for risk/benefit. Greg did not understand why I could not give Jill standard treatment plus the additional therapy; he knew another patient in my office who was receiving the "additional therapy drug" who was not on a clinical trial. I explained that my other patient had advanced cancer for which the additional therapy was approved but it was not approved for Jill's stage of cancer. Giving therapies to patients before they are approved is risky, as clinical trials not only evaluate the reduction in risk of recurrence but also the negative aspects of new therapies, such as side effects and complications. The only way Jill could receive the additional therapy was by participating in a clinical trial, and then only if she was randomized to the investigational arm of the study.

After one more night to sleep on their decision, Jill and Greg signed the informed consent. The following Monday, after all necessary tests were completed per the clinical trial requirements, treatment was begun. Blood tests, additional X-rays, and a test to measure Jill's heart function had been performed, and fortunately, no abnormalities were detected. Jill was randomized to receive the investigational additional therapy as well as the standard chemotherapy.

For my patients like Jill and Greg and their families, the final treatment decision generates a collective sigh of relief. Positive attitudes usually prevail over the fears and anxieties of treatment side effects once treatment begins. However, patients at this point usually have new questions. I will address the most common questions in Section 3.

# SECTION 3

# More Questions

## Introduction

The shock of a cancer diagnosis and the wealth of information presented to patients in the weeks and months immediately following the pronouncement "you have cancer" are numbing. Often, as patients become accustomed to the routine of adjuvant therapy, they wish to discuss many issues that the care team began to address before initiating treatment. They also have new concerns about diet, exercise, sexuality, and living with a cancer diagnosis. In this section, in addition to the above concerns, I discuss some of the more common themes my patients ask about: the issues of CANCER PREVENTION, TREATMENT SURVEILLANCE, and CANCER RELAPSE. We begin with the question next asked by Greg: Wouldn't Jill benefit from ALTERNATIVE THERAPIES?

# Chapter Five

# Alternative Therapies

Shortly after initiating Jill's treatment, Greg called regarding an article in the newspaper that praised a new wonder drug for breast cancer. The "wonder drug" discussion raised the broader question of how a patient and their supportive family members remain sane amidst the endless reports of breakthroughs, miracles, and cures. There is no easy answer. In my observation, the key to sanity is found in a patient's trust in the integrity of his or her caregivers and faith in his or her own judgment. All patients will reach a line in the sand when they have to decide on treatment. Only by believing that they have performed adequate due diligence and by trusting their caregivers' recommendations can that decision be made without regret. Jill and Greg went through such a process. I believed they had a foundation of faith and trust that would keep them sane in the coming months and years.

Jill also raised the possibility of pursuing alternative therapy. Thankfully, before embarking on such an initiative, she consulted with me. I thought some definitions were needed to help us structure the discussion. UNCONVENTIONAL, ALTERNATIVE, or COMPLEMENTARY THERAPIES encompass a broad spectrum of practices and beliefs and are, therefore, very difficult to define. What is common to these therapies is that they do not conform with the beliefs or standards of the conventional mainstream medical establishment or accepted standard of care. These standards can also be culturally dependent, which may create further confusion, i.e., traditional Chinese medicine is considered unconventional in the United States, whereas it is a standard practice in China. Also, with unconventional therapies, their proof of effectiveness is most often conveyed through personal anecdote rather than stringent, evidence-based criteria reached through multiphase clinical research.

Unconventional therapies may be subdivided into complementary therapies and alternative therapies. Complementary therapies can be further categorized as spiritual, psychological, nutritional, and physical. Meditation, relaxation, imaging, prayer, massage, and dietary supplements are just a few of the interventions in the broad class of complementary therapies. These approaches to healing are not in conflict with conventional Western medicine; rather, in most cases, they can be effectively integrated into standard medical practice. Alternative therapies, as the name implies, are not intended to be integrated into conventional therapy; rather, they are offered as a complete therapy intended to be used instead of the standard of care. Unproven by evidence-based criteria, pharmacologic treatments comprise the bulk of alternative therapies. These therapies are particularly susceptible to quackery, and false and excessive claims and high-profit motives are common.

The increased interest in and attractiveness of unconventional therapies are understandable. The technologic and frequently impersonal nature of modern medicine leaves patients feeling lost and empty. Insensitive, hurried interactions with physicians often result in patients feeling helpless, out of control, and ignored. The confusing jargon and statistics further alienate the patient and family. Finally, the cold, hard truth of some cancer diagnoses and the limited effectiveness of some conventional standard therapies may foster hopelessness. Unconventional medicine, on the other hand, is perceived as natural, simpler, nontoxic, and more understandable. Its practitioners are viewed as more caring and their approach more holistic. The absence of data eliminates the difficult discussions of toxicity, response, and survival probability.

Greg asked, "How does one evaluate and choose an unconventional approach to healing?" There are a few guidelines that I suggest my patients follow. First, avoid any practitioner of any unconventional (or for that matter, mainstream) method who is evasive. People who practice healing techniques that they believe in will want to share them with your other doctors, not hide them. Second, avoid treatments that are touted to work only if you stop your traditional treatments. Especially with cancer treatment, we need to take advantage of all treatments that may help. Third, avoid practitioners who have exclusive access to the cure but will not tell anyone what it is. Practitioners who truly believe in what they are doing want to share their successes. Fourth, beware of the motivations of the people making recommendations.

It is unusual for natural healing techniques to be very expensive. If an exclusive treatment is being suggested and is very expensive, examine the motivations of the prescriber. Be aware that most unconventional therapies are not covered by insurance, given the absence of supporting data from well-designed clinical trials. Finally, pick an unconventional therapy that you feel good enough about to discuss with your physician. Your participation in restoring or maintaining your health is absolutely essential. The success of many alternative treatments depends in great part on your belief in the potential of the therapy to improve your health. If you truly believe in the therapy, be willing to discuss it not only with your family and friends, but also with your physician.

Jill and Greg seemed comfortable with my response. I told them that if they came across a particularly appealing complementary treatment, they should bring it to my attention for discussion. As I was about to leave the room, I noticed that Jill appeared uneasy. I asked again if she was comfortable with her treatment decision. She said that this was not what was troubling her. She said she worried about her daughter's, sister's, and mother's risk of breast cancer, even though her cancer was found not to be hereditary. I told her that much would change before her daughter would be at risk and there were steps her mother and sister could take right now to reduce their risk of getting cancer.

# Chapter Six

# Prevention

S trategies have recently been designed that may help to prevent first and subsequent breast cancers. These strategies include lifestyle modifications, genetic testing, surgery, and medication. The two most significant life style issues that may play an important role in prevention are diet and exercise. Dietary fats, alcohol, sedentary behavior, and obesity are all being actively investigated as possible factors that increase the risk of cancer, and not just breast cancer. Studies of both men and women have suggested that three or more hours of vigorous exercise a week may significantly reduce the risk of developing cancer. Alcohol's effect on the liver may increase circulating estrogen levels, creating a biochemical basis for its relationship to breast cancer.

Dietary fats have been implicated in cancer ever since the observation that cancer is more frequent in westernized countries that consume a diet richer in animal foods, meat and dairy. Fats are specifically related to breast cancer because countries with very low breast cancer incidence—for example Japan—also have very low-fat diets. Unfortunately, this remains unproven, as research has failed to follow up these epidemiological findings with rigorous tests of diets as low in fat (as a percentage of total calorie intake) as those observed in Asia and Africa. The average American consumes approximately 35% of their total calories from fat. Dietary fats are not the only area of concern. Total calorie intake and alcohol consumption have also been implicated in breast cancers.

The role of vitamins and minerals in cancer prevention remains highly controversial. However, in 2008, scientists from the University of Toronto made a presentation at the American Society of Clinical Oncology suggesting breast cancer patients might fare worse if they had low levels of vitamin D in their blood at the time of their diagnosis. Women with the lowest levels of vitamin D (i.e., vitamin D deficient) had nearly double the risk of their disease progressing, and a 73% greater risk of death compared to women with adequate vitamin D. The findings were statistically significant and were not affected by factors including age, weight, tumor stage or tumor grade. The study author cautions that her findings are preliminary and need to be repeated in other studies before firm conclusions about vitamin D and breast cancer can be drawn.

A great deal of research has also been focused on developing drugs that can prevent cancer. The preventative treatment of cancer with a drug is called CHEMOPREVENTION. Two drugs, tamoxifen (Nolvadex), and Evista (raloxifene), have now been approved for the chemoprevention of breast cancer. The Study of Tamoxifen and Raloxifene, referred to as the "STAR Trial," demonstrated that Evista, like tamoxifen, can reduce the incidence of new breast cancers in high-risk women. Unlike Tamoxifen, Evista is indicated for use in post-menopausal women only. Earlier research suggested that breast cancer incidence may be reduced by as much as 50% with medications that interfere with estrogen. This suggestion was initially confirmed by a trial comparing the preventative effects of tamoxifen to a sugar pill placebo. Proof of tamoxifen's benefit led to the STAR Trial, which in turn led to an ongoing trial evaluating the preventative benefits of aromatase inhibitors. Who should receive chemoprevention, with what drug, and for how long remains to be established, but multidisciplinary consensus conferences using evidence-based clinical research are beginning to shed light on this area.

A community survey found that 23% of women expressed interest in breast cancer chemoprevention. Worry about breast cancer was the strongest predictor of interest, but there was no association between interest and objectively estimated personal risk. Smokers were nearly twice as likely as nonsmokers to express interest in chemoprevention. Mortality rates underscore the irony of this finding. Of 1,000 50-year-old women who smoke, four will die of breast cancer in the ensuing 10 years, 13 will die of heart attacks, 10 of lung cancer, and six of stroke. So the women who were twice as likely to take a breast cancer prevention pill were ten times more likely to die from smoking-related disease than from breast cancer. Such surveys reinforce the need to determine who are the most appropriate candidates for chemoprevention and the need to greatly improve health education.

On the basis of its review of the evidence, the U.S. Preventive Services Task Force (USPSTF) recommends against widespread use of chemoprevention for patients with a low or average risk for breast cancer. The USPSTF recommends discussing chemoprevention with selected patients at high risk for breast cancer and at low risk for the most serious adverse events (endometrial cancer, pulmonary embolus, and stroke induced by tamoxifen), (see Table 2-1, page 33).

The current evidence leaves many questions unanswered. Do chemoprevention agents prevent cancer or treat very early cases? How long does the effect of lowered incidence of breast cancer persist after taking a chemopreventive drug for five years? Will breast cancer cells develop resistance to tamoxifen? Together, these issues beg the big question: Does chemoprevention reduce breast cancer and all-cause mortality, and, if so, by how much?

The USPSTF recommendations present two serious challenges for clinicians. First, clinicians must respond to the misinformed and mitigate the worry that may cloud perspective and create demand for chemoprevention when the potential harms may far exceed the benefits. Second, clinicians must identify and engage the uninformed for whom, because of their risk profile and personal preference, chemoprevention holds potential promise.

Risk estimation and communication are at the center of both challenges. The most frequently used risk assessment tool, the GAIL MODEL, estimates the five-year incidence of breast cancer for a patient on the basis of the woman's age, number of first-degree relatives with breast cancer, no pregnancies or age at birth of first child, number of breast biopsies, pathologic diagnosis of atypical hyperplasia, and age at onset of first menstrual cycle. For women whose worry results from an exaggerated perception of risks, such estimates may provide reassurance.

Making fateful decisions that depend on medical science as well as highly personal judgments about how future illness will affect quality of life is difficult at best. Neither doctor nor patient can do it alone. With breast cancer chemoprevention, clinicians and patients need to understand the limits of what we know and what we can control about the future. Women and doctors who work at making good decisions together will be far more likely to make the best use of what current medical science has to offer.

After much thought, Jill and her mom decided that five years of a SERM might not be the best choice for her mom or sister. We all agreed that it was appropriate for both to continue annual mammography and for her mom to continue her daily two-mile walk. Jill's mom also agreed to limit her wine consumption to the weekends and increase the amount of fruits and vegetables in her diet. She would ask her doctor to check a vitamin D level at her next visit.

# Chapter Seven

# Advanced Cancer

Jill and Greg had raised the "what if" question about relapse. I had hoped to avoid this discussion as it can be unpleasant to talk about treatment failure, and, in any case, it was unlikely given Jill's probability of cure. Occasionally, cancer will recur only in the preserved breast, axilla, or chest wall. In these cases, it is referred to as a LOCAL RECURRENCE and is likely curable. However, most relapses are systemic, which means they are metastases. Metastases are rarely cured. I could not think of a gentle way to approach metastatic cancer, so I decided to detour for a bit, beginning the discussion with locally advanced cancer, a subject that I neglected in our earlier discussion.

## Locally Advanced High-Risk Breast Cancer

I have previously focused on women who undergo surgical removal of the breast tumor and subsequent adjuvant therapy to destroy micrometastasis, thus reducing the risk of relapse. These women are said to have LOCALIZED breast cancer, and consensus guidelines offer reasonable clarity in the approach to management. I now discuss the woman with LOCALLY ADVANCED breast cancer: either a large breast mass (greater than 5 cm) or palpable axiliary lymph nodes at presentation or a breast mass that involves the overlying skin or is fixed to the underlying chest wall. Guidelines to direct management of these patients is less clear, and thus, I will share where current research is leading us.

A woman who presents with locally advanced breast cancer may benefit from a new treatment approach: chemotherapy before surgery. This approach, called neoadjuvant chemotherapy (or primary systemic therapy), attempts to make the cancer more accessible to breast conservation surgery. Unlike the use of chemotherapy in the adjuvant setting—which treats possible micrometastases—the effect of neoadjuvant chemotherapy can be directly observed as the tumor shrinks, remains stable, or grows. Recent studies demonstrate growth of tumor during treatment in less than 10% of neoadjuvantly treated patients. Neoadjuvant chemotherapy demonstrates the effectiveness of chemotherapy (chemo sensitivity) and shrinks tumors, permitting breast conservation. These benefits as well as the hope that such an approach may increase the cure rate in this high-risk population are making the neoadjuvant approach increasingly popular among physicians and patients. Regardless of the approach, the successful treatment of women with locally advanced breast cancer requires the coordinated efforts of surgical, radiation, and medical oncologists. All three treatment modalities are needed to optimize the cure rate.

## Metastatic Breast Cancer

When the cancer has spread beyond the breast and regional lymph nodes it is referred to as metastatic. Even when the cancer is found to be metastatic, all hope is not lost as some patients with metastatic cancer can be cured. For the many who cannot be cured, advances in treatment are making metastatic breast cancer more like a chronic disease than the death sentence it was once considered. Most oncologists subdivide metastatic cancer into two categories, OLIGOMETASTATIC and DIFFUSE METASTATIC. Oligomets are usually small, limited in number and found in a single site of organ metastatic disease, such as the liver or lung. Advances in imaging technology and treatment permit these patients to be treated with CURATIVE INTENT. Combining systemic treatment with surgery, radiation and INTERVENTIONAL RADIOLOGY can often render patients cancer free and sometimes cured.

Despite all of the described methods to screen, diagnose, and adjuvantly treat breast cancer when it is localized, 25% of all breast cancer patients still die from their disease because the cancer diffusely metastasizes to the vital organs: lung, liver, and brain. They also may suffer from cancer involvement of bone, lymph nodes, and skin, and recurrences may develop in the chest wall of the originally involved breast. Breast cancer in this situation is rarely curable, but a great deal can be done to diminish symptoms, improve quality of life, and prolong life. Therapy intended not to cure but to improve the quality of life is called PALLIATIVE.

The evaluation and management of patients with diffuse metastatic disease either at initial presentation or after relapse can be performed in a similar way to those with curable cancer. Unfortunately, since cure is rare in diffuse metastatic disease, the most important goals are survival time and quality of life. I recommend using the percentage of women alive at one, two, three, and five years after treatment as a meaningful measure of treatment effectiveness. Survival may be the ultimate goal of treatment, but the care of the patient with diffuse and often symptomatic metastatic disease is complicated by the need to manage disease-related symptoms. Before survival can be considered, suffering must be palliated. The ability of a treatment to palliate symptoms is often measured as its response rate. Response may be more important than survival in a suffering patient. Outcomes, such as one-year survival and clinical response, are most commonly presented in relative terms but can also be presented as absolute impact using the 100-patient method described previously.

Because all treatments have side effects, palliative therapy demands a uniquely candid discussion of goals and objectives between the oncologist and patient. Expressions such as "watch and wait," "the cure may be worse than the disease," and "win the battle but lose the war" are attempts by oncologists to explain to the patient that when it comes to palliative therapy, more is not always better. The main objective in palliative therapy is maximal preservation of quality of life, not maximal tumor shrinkage, unless shrinkage (response) has been proven to impact directly the quality of life or survival.

# Chapter Eight

# Posttreatment Surveillance and Supportive Care

Consensus panels continue to recommend posttreatment follow-up for women with Stages I, II, and III breast cancer. Follow-up should include performance of routine history and physical examinations, mammography, and, if treated with tamoxifen, pelvic examination if the uterus is present. Surveillance may be as frequent as every three months in the first few years after diagnosis or as infrequent as annually beyond five years from diagnosis. However, surveillance is recommended for the life of the patient as both late relapse of breast cancer and late adverse effects of treatments have been reported as many as 30 years after diagnosis. Routine surveillance by BONE SCAN and CT SCAN are not recommended, to the dismay of most patients. Unfortunately, neither of these approaches has been proven effective. Similar to the screening tests that were discussed earlier, for a surveillance to be effective it must be proven to be both sensitive and specific. Insensitive tests will miss abnormalities. Sensitive tests that are not specific will reveal abnormalities that are not related to the cancer, often leading to more tests, procedures, and anxiety that may not only be not helpful but seriously harmful. Researchers continue to evaluate new technologies that might enhance the ability to both diagnose and predict relapse. PET scanning and other imaging, genetic and routine blood chemistry testing such as the CA 27-29 and CA 15-3 are still considered investigational. Genomics and proteinomics as well as microarray testing hold the greatest promise but may not be commercially available for years.

# Epilogue

During the next few months, Jill and Greg slowly settled into the reality of her therapy. The first six weeks were the toughest, as she experienced reconstruction-related pain, suffered the indignity of hair loss, and dealt with the side effects of chemotherapy. The emotional impact of her treatment overwhelmed her more than the physical effects. It's not easy to confront mortality at any age, certainly not at thirty-seven. Greg and the rest of her family's doting and well-intentioned support only worsened her sense of vulnerability. She became clinically depressed. I recommended counseling and an antidepressant. She agreed.

Three months into systemic therapy, Jill seemed to turn a corner. Counseling and antidepressant therapy were helping. Her treatment tolerance improved and the reconstruction-related pain resolved. She was mostly bothered by a sense of fatigue that she likened to that experienced during her pregnancies. Now, Jill was finally able to look at herself in the mirror without becoming ill and crying. She was beginning to feel that the worst was behind her and that life might return to normal.

Near the conclusion of chemotherapy, she experienced an emotional setback. I thought she would approach the day of her last treatment with elation, but surprisingly, she seemed depressed. Our conversation uncovered a growing emotional dependency on her active treatment as her protection against a cancer relapse. I explained that her chemotherapy had accomplished what was intended and that it was time to advance her treatment to antiestrogen therapy. The five years of oral tamoxifen, which she was about to initiate, was as important to her cure as was the chemotherapy. She started taking tamoxifen, remaining upbeat and resilient despite the severe hot flashes that would continue for three months.

Two years from that fateful day when the words "you have cancer" forever changed their lives, Jill, Greg, Amy, and Josh were a happy and healthy suburban family once again. Selective memory and the healing effects of time proved to be an effective salve to the physical and emotional wounds inflicted by her cancer diagnosis. Like millions of Americans, Jill and Greg found that they had what it takes to be survivors.

M y only remaining question as I close this discussion of breast cancer is on the lighter side: Did I have what it takes to survive a classroom of fifteen second-graders? As you recall, I left Daniel's room contemplating what kind of cancer machine to demonstrate and what memento I could leave for the class. I decided Legos were a more-than-adequate prop for my presentation. After all, a two-ton linear accelerator would not fit through the classroom door.

What to give second-graders was a bigger challenge. I contacted Ken, a pharmaceutical representative, who said he could donate some promotional fanny-packs. His company's marketing department developed a fanny-pack filled with exercise-related items including a water bottle, towel, and stopwatch to create the notion that fatigue-busting drug for cancer patients could get them back into exercising. I was elated as I realized that a fanny-pack bulging with all this junk would be the best give-away that any parent could have.

The day arrived, and before curious eyes, Daniel and I entered the classroom with Legos and fanny-packs. Daniel's teacher brought the class to order, then asked Daniel to introduce me.

Daniel's introduction was the essence of brevity. "This is my dad."

The kids were great. They were attentive, well behaved and—believe it or not—interested. Upon the conclusion of my demonstration, the teacher asked the students if they had any questions. The hands shot up. I was overwhelmed at the response and pointed to a boy in the back row. He asked, "What's the best thing about your job?" I said, "It's nice to be able to help people." More hands soared. "What's the worst part of your job?" I explained that I'm not able to make all the sick people who see me feel better. More hands went up, and my head was swelling to the size of a watermelon. "What's the best part of your job?" I said, "In addition to helping people I get to come home at night and play with Daniel." I looked at Daniel; he was beaming. More hands. "What's the worst part of your job?" I may be gullible, but I'm not stupid. "Is there anyone with a question other than what is the best or worst part of my job?" I was praying that just one hand would still be up, but none were. They were all shills asking the questions planted by their teacher.

Once again, I was humbled by children. I thanked the teacher and said goodbye to the class. As I left, I looked over my shoulder to see Daniel grinning ear to ear.

# Appendix

## This section will answer questions frequently asked by cancer survivors.

### Remission, Cure & Recurrence

When cancer treatment is complete, the first question most survivors ask is: "Am I cured?" The term **cure** means to heal or restore health. In general, it means there are no signs of cancer in the body. **Remission** is a decrease or disappearance of signs or symptoms of cancer. A **complete remission** means that all signs or symptoms of cancer have disappeared and it is undetectable, although cancer may still be in the body. **Recurrence** is when cancer returns after a period of time during which it cannot be detected. Medical oncologists rarely use the term "**cure,**" although it is the word most survivors most want to hear. If you have questions about these terms or how to interpret them for your particular situation, ask your medical oncologist for assistance.

## Q: Do I need to see my oncologist after I finish treatment?

**A:** All cancer survivors will require scheduled follow-up care with their oncologist. The frequency of follow-up will be determined by your specific type of cancer and the treatment you received. Many people will keep their ports for at least one year after treatment, requiring maintenance on a monthly basis. Follow-up appointments with your medical oncologist are generally scheduled every three to four months for the first two years after completing treatment. For three to five years after treatment, your oncologist will see you every six to 12 months. Once you have reached the five-year mark, your follow-up will be scheduled annually or your care may be turned over to your primary care physician. Depending on the type of cancer, laboratory studies, radiographic studies, and/or biopsies may be ordered.

## Q: What do I do if I have a problem?

**A:** Although you will have scheduled follow-up appointments, do not wait until a scheduled appointment if you experience new symptoms. These symptoms may include unexplained fever, night sweats, weight loss, pain, new lumps or bumps, fatigue, bleeding, increased bruising, new cough, changes in breathing, chest pain, bowel pattern changes, trouble sleeping, sexual problems, or other problems which have developed since completing treatment.

At your follow-up appointment, provide an updated list of medications you are taking, including all vitamins and herbal preparations. It is a good idea to bring all of your medications along for review by the health care provider. Discuss any changes in your family's medical history, particularly if someone has been diagnosed with cancer.

## Q: My doctor says I'm in remission, but I go to bed every night thinking about the cancer.

**A:** Fear of cancer returning is almost always present for someone who has had cancer. Loss of control, anxiety, and depression are common feelings after cancer treatment. Support groups and professional counselors are available through your health care provider and in your community to help you cope with these feelings and symptoms. Through support and/ or counseling, you can find new ways to deal with fears of cancer returning by accepting what has happened, recognizing that there are some things you cannot control, and finding some things you can control.

## Q: Will I ever resume a normal sleep pattern?

**A:** When it comes to sleeping, quality counts—not quantity. Try to go to bed and get up at the same time each day. Avoid long naps as this may be disrupting your natural sleep cycle at night. If you have trouble falling asleep, try eating a snack with tryptophan. A turkey or tuna sandwich on wheat, a glass of warm milk, or a bowl of hot oatmeal made with milk all contain tryptophan. Avoid alcohol, caffeine, and heavy meals in the evening. Your bed has only two purposes: sleep and you know the other. Do not use your bed as a lounge chair; don't eat in bed.

# Q: Why do I feel so tired?

**A:** Despite the number of people who suffer from fatigue during cancer treatment (90% or more), the causes and best treatments are still unclear. Often, cancer centers may not address fatigue simply because they aren't aware of successful ways to manage it. At least 30% of cancer patients report fatigue lasting months to years beyond treatment. If you are experiencing fatigue, you are not alone.

If you suffer from ongoing fatigue, ask for help. Remember, quality of life matters. Fatigue will likely impact your quality of life the most.

## Steps to managing your fatigue:

Evaluate your current diet, vitamins, and fluid intake.

- Eat enough calories to meet your energy needs. Calories from carbohydrates are our main energy source.

- Drink two liters per day of fluids such as water, decaffeinated drinks, and juices.

- Take a multivitamin daily.

- To help repair and rebuild the body's tissues, include protein at every meal and snack, preferably from plant-based foods. If you're trying to lose weight, use low-fat protein sources such as lean meats, skim milk, egg whites, and low-fat cheeses.

- If you have problems that affect eating, such as taste changes or chronic diarrhea, discuss these with your health care team or a Registered Dietitian (RD) in your area.

## Exercise.

- Work toward a goal of 15–30 minutes of activity most days of the week. Exercise limits the breakdown of muscle tissue, which also helps decrease your overall feeling of tiredness.

- Add weight training twice per week to rebuild muscle tone and keep bones strong. Women with a history of breast cancer can particularly benefit from strength training.

### Discuss your current medications with your physician, nurse, dietitian, or pharmacist.

- Medications for pain, high blood pressure, depression, nausea, and allergies can all cause fatigue.

- You may be able to stop some medications now that your treatment is done. Talk with your physician about which medications can be discontinued.

### Discuss lab results with your physician, nurse, or other provider.

- Untreated anemia can cause fatigue.

- Low electrolyte (magnesium, potassium, sodium) levels, due to vomiting or diarrhea, can make you tired.

- Vitamin deficiencies can cause fatigue.

- If you received radiation to your head or neck, your thyroid may have been affected. Ask your physician to check your thyroid levels.

### See your primary care physician to help evaluate any other illnesses you may have.

- Do you have another health condition that could be causing fatigue? Lung disease, congestive heart failure, thyroid dysfunction, and uncontrolled diabetes can all make you feel tired.

## Q: What do I do if I have pain?

A: Pain can interfere with your appetite, energy, and sleep. Be aware that pain medications can make you tired and constipated. Talk with your health care team about pain treatments that may not make you sleepy. Pain medications, which were appropriate during cancer treatment, may no longer be needed. Pain due to chemotherapy treatment may linger for months after treatment is complete. However this should gradually diminish. You may need an evaluation by a pain management specialist if pain continues more than three months beyond treatment.

## Q: Sometimes I feel anxious but I don't think I'm depressed.

A: If you think you may be experiencing anxiety or depression, don't ignore it. Talk with a friend, pastor, or family member, or ask your physician for a referral to a counselor or psychologist. Symptoms of anxiety include shortness of breath, sweating, excessive worrying, rapid heart beat, nervousness, and difficulty concentrating. Symptoms of depression include decreased interest in your usual activities, sleepiness or sleeping too much, feelings of sadness and hopelessness, isolating yourself, irritability, and feeling tired even when you've had quality sleep. If these symptoms occur more than two or three times a week, it is important to talk with your physician. Ensure that you are managing stressors—consider a support group, exercise, or other activities you enjoy.

## Q: I know I'm not crazy. It's been three months since I finished chemo and my mind is still in a fog.

A: Cognitive changes (changes in thinking) are common after certain cancer treatments. People typically report problems in the areas of memory and concentration. This experience is frequently referred to as "chemobrain" by cancer survivors. It can sometimes feel like mental fuzziness or a slowed-down thinking process. Often the mind, not just the body, is tired from all that you have been through. If you are experiencing these symptoms, tell your physician and provide specific examples to help them assess the situation, such as: "I can't concentrate on my work," or "I forget where my keys are and I can't seem to think through the steps in order to find them." Fortunately, there are steps you can take to combat "chemobrain." Here are some specific examples of ways to both increase concentration and improve your memory:

- Eliminate distractions such as cell phones, TVs, and other background noise when you are trying to concentrate.

- Make sure that you get adequate rest and good nutrition. Lack of sleep and hunger can make concentrating even more difficult.

- Studies have shown that stimulating the mind through crossword puzzles and board games, decreasing alcohol consumption, getting enough sleep, and decreasing stress help to restore a person's memory and thinking processes.

- Keep a pad of paper or notebook on hand. Use it to write down reminders and any distracting thoughts so you can concentrate on your task at hand.

- Break your tasks into manageable parts. You will begin to feel more confident if you see that you are making progress.

- Take time to get away from your tasks. Frequent breaks may help you clear your mind and come back to your task fresh and invigorated.

- Think about the conditions that help you to concentrate. Are you at your best with soft music playing? With a cup of coffee and good lighting? With a clean desk? In the morning or evening?

- Organize the places you most frequently use so that things are in predictable spaces.

- If memory seems to be the most difficult challenge, state things aloud, such as "I am placing my keys on the kitchen counter." Hearing things aloud gives your mind another clue when you're trying to remember.

- If you feel strong enough, take a yoga or meditation class. Try painting or poetry writing. Restorative activities are more important now than ever before as you transition to cancer survivorship.

- Share these symptoms with others. People often report that they are afraid to admit that they are having difficulty with memory and concentration. If your employer, friends, or family know that this is a normal symptom, they will likely be more understanding and may even help you develop routines that will reinforce your efforts.

Keep in mind that you are trying to retrain your mind to concentrate and remember more efficiently. It's important to be patient with the process but also to know that concentration is learned and must be practiced just like any other skill.

## Q: It's been two months since my last treatment and I physically feel fine, but I have no sexual desire and my husband is becoming concerned.

A: Sexuality is a complex issue that is affected not only by life and relationships prior to cancer, but the physical and emotional issues between you and your partner. It involves not only intercourse, but all the feelings and actions associated with loving and caring for someone, including hugging, caressing, and holding hands.

Survivors often feel that they are alone in their experiences, but 40–100 percent of survivors have some complaints or concerns about sexual issues after treatment. Functional damage to tissues and muscles from cancer therapies, fatigue, pain, and fear can affect not only the physical aspects of sex, but also the enjoyment of the sexual relationship as a whole. Survivors and their partners need to learn to communicate clearly, make accommodations, and plan ahead to make sexual relations as comfortable and stress-free as possible.

After treatment, a normal sex life may be different for individuals and the key requirement is that it should be pleasurable for both partners. Frequency and desire can vary after treatment just as they did prior to treatment. Talking to each other about wants and desires will help partners to develop a close and intimate relationship. As other aspects of your life begin to return to normal, sexual desires and activities should also return but may be different than before.

Fatigue resulting from surgery, chemotherapy, and radiation is a common complaint among cancer survivors. Being too tired for sexual activity is very normal both during and after cancer treatment. Cuddling, hugging, and other physical expressions may be less exhausting and still provide the warmth and closeness desired by the survivor and his or her partner. Be aware that fatigue and lack of sexual desire are two warning signs of depression. If they continue, you may want to seek professional help.

Pain, or fear of pain, is an issue that many survivors face. Pain can be caused by physical changes due to surgery, radiation, and some cancer treatment related drugs. It is important to understand that sexual activity should never be painful. If pain does occur while engaging in sex, communicate to your partner that you need to stop, consult your physician, and perhaps seek some additional help. When sexual experiences are painful or do not go well for any reason, there is a greater risk for sexual difficulty in the future. There are many products such as lubricating creams and gels (e.g., Astroglide, K-Y gel, and Replens), dilators, or other prescription appliances that can make intercourse more comfortable. Prescription medications which enhance sexual performance in men may be indicated. Sometimes, changing to a different position for intercourse will eliminate the pain and make intimacy pleasurable again.

Fears about body image, desirability, and performance are common concerns for cancer survivors. Frequently they feel ashamed and embarrassed to talk with their partners and instead worry silently, making them appear more withdrawn and less interested in sex. An open conversation that is initiated by the partner may help the survivor to open up, express their concerns, and receive reassurance. If it is too difficult to start a conversation on this topic, either partner can try writing their feelings in the form of a note. It is most important for both partners to be as comfortable as possible about sharing their feelings and their bodies with each other in order to achieve sexual satisfaction.

Learning to develop realistic expectations for sexual performance is an important step for success. Learning to accept, appreciate, and honor your body will enable self-image and confidence to grow.

A warm, loving, and equally enjoyable sexual relationship is available to you and your partner as long as you are willing and able to be open with each other, work through difficulties, and, if necessary, seek professional help.

Survivors and their partners may find it difficult to talk with their physician about their sexual difficulties and may be more comfortable talking with a therapist specializing in sexual issues.

A sex therapist is a physician, nurse, or social worker who has been educated to treat sexual dysfunction. The best way to get a reputable referral is through your physician or gynecologist. Most will talk with you on the phone prior to an appointment regarding their experience treating cancer patients. For help, contact the American Association of Sex Educators, Counselors, and Therapists at (319) 895-8407.

## Q: Ever since my diagnosis I've had such a short fuse. What can I do?

**A:** You probably experienced a variety of emotions when you were first diagnosed with cancer and again when you underwent treatment. Cancer survivors often experience a new set of emotions when cancer treatment is complete. As you move forward with your life, you may feel:

- Fear of the cancer returning

- Your priorities changing

- Your family responsibilities changing

- Your spiritual beliefs changing

- Pressure to return to your daily life as it was before cancer

Scheduling tests, developing treatment plans, and coping with the side effects of cancer treatment may delay your adjustment to returning to your own life. Although you have finished cancer treatment, you will be left with a great deal of emotions that were never recognized. Family, friends, co-workers, and even you may assume that because treatment is finished you will go back to being the same person you were before cancer. You may also have a new set of emotions when moving back into your routine schedule. Expect a slow, gradual adjustment to your family role or role in the workplace. You may find that your definition of normal has changed. You may still be coping with treatment side effects such as tiredness, nerve damage, difficulty sleeping, pain, nausea, or others. These may take time to improve.

Feeling angry, isolated, and uncertain is common after cancer treatment, even if you never felt those emotions before. Many people join support groups at this phase in their lives to get help with these feelings. At cancer support group meetings, you will find that you are not alone and others share your same feelings and fears. Rather than trying to forget the experience of cancer, it is a more realistic goal to move forward with your life while still recognizing cancer's impact on you. Some people find it rewarding and comforting to become a mentor to other cancer patients through volunteer work or by developing support groups of their own. Recognizing that you are a changed person from this major life experience can better prepare you to live your life to the fullest.

## Q: Everyday I read another article in the paper about what to eat to stay cancer free. I'm so confused.

A: One of the most important lifestyle changes you can make during the time following treatment is to improve the foods that you eat on a daily basis. The powerful effects of maintaining a healthy diet will aid in healing from your treatment and its side effects, can prevent the recurrence of cancer, and may prevent other chronic diseases like diabetes and heart disease. Your goal is to center your food choices around plant foods like fruits, vegetables, whole grains, and legumes. These guidelines are intended to help you begin eating healthier every day so you can rebuild a strong, powerful body that fights disease.

## Eat seven or more servings of fruits and vegetables every day.

**One serving of fruits and vegetables equals:**

1 cup raw, ½ cup cooked or canned, ¼ cup dried fruit, 1 small piece of fruit, or 4-6 oz. 100% juice

Include many colorful fruits and vegetables in your meals and snacks, such as carrots, dried cranberries, or apples. Limit the amount of fried vegetables, such as french fries, onion rings, and fried okra. By choosing more fruits and vegetables, you will increase your intake of phytochemicals (plant nutrients) and antioxidants, which help keep your cells strong and free of damage.

**Below are some examples of phytochemicals and antioxidants, along with their food sources:**

- Beta-carotene—carrots, cooked pumpkin, red bell peppers, spinach, kale, sweet potatoes or yams, cantaloupe, mango

- Vitamin C—guava fruit, brussels sprouts, strawberries, papaya, grapefruit sections, broccoli, orange juice, kale

- Vitamin E—sunflower seeds, almonds, wheat germ, cooked soybeans, barley

- Selenium—brazil nuts, tofu, shrimp, shitake mushrooms

- Anthocyanins—blueberries, strawberries, red cabbage, plums, cherries, raspberries

- Multiple—(Cruciferous vegetables) bok choy, broccoli, brussels sprouts, cabbage, cauliflower, collard, turnip, and mustard greens, radishes, turnips

- Allium—garlic, leeks, onions, scallions, shallots, chives

- Lycopene—processed tomato products (salsa, canned tomatoes, tomato juice, spaghetti sauce, sun dried tomatoes), watermelon, pink grapefruit

# If you drink alcohol, limit your intake.

If you drink alcohol, limit to two drinks per day for men, one drink per day for women.

(1 drink = 12 oz. beer, 5 oz. wine, or 1.5 oz. of 80 proof liquor)

Alcohol intake may increase the risk of cancer. Therefore, cancer survivors should be cautious regarding alcohol intake.

# Choose whole grains and plant proteins for adequate fiber intake.

Your goal is to eat 25–35 grams of dietary fiber per day. Replace white bread, spaghetti, and white rice with whole-wheat bread, whole-wheat pasta, and brown rice. Read your nutrition labels carefully and choose grains with three or more grams of fiber per serving. Also, three days per week, try to replace red meat and poultry at meals with dried beans, nuts, or soybean-based foods. (A cautionary note with soy: If the cancer was estrogen receptor positive, consult a dietician.)

1 oz. meat is equivalent to ½ cup beans, ¼ cup nuts, 1 oz. texturized vegetable protein.

If you choose at least three servings of whole grains, two fruits, and three servings of vegetables daily, you should easily meet your daily requirement of 25–35 grams of fiber.

# Choose a low-fat meal plan that focuses on plant-based fats and limits saturated and trans fat.

The kinds of fat you eat are also important. Focus on eating, in moderate amounts, plant-based fats (monounsaturated and polyunsaturated fats). Choose olive, peanut, or canola oil over margarine and butter. Choose avocados or olives to flavor sandwiches instead of mayonnaise or cheese. Eat foods high in Omega-3 fatty acids (a polyunsaturated fat) such as salmon, trout, tuna, swordfish, flaxseed and flaxseed oil, canola and soybean oils, walnuts, and wheat germ. Bake, stew, or steam foods instead of frying. Choose low-fat or non-fat dairy foods.

# Choose fresh foods as often as possible.

Your goal is to limit processed foods and salt in your overall diet. Limit your salt intake by eating less pickled foods, canned soups and vegetables, soy sauce, Chinese cuisine, fast foods, and frozen dinners. Limit salted, smoked, cured, and processed meats such as bacon, ham, pepperoni, sausage, Spam, luncheon and canned meats, hot dogs, and jerky. When possible, prepare these foods at home so that you control how much salt you use in your cooking. Use pepper, fresh or dried spices, and herbs instead of salt in preparing your meals. Choose and purchase fresh fish, poultry, and meat alternatives such as soy/veggie burgers more often. Select lean cuts of red meat and poultry and smaller portion sizes. Prepare meats by baking, steaming, poaching, or braising.

## Q: First my doctor was concerned about my weight loss, but now he is getting on my case for weight gain.

A: Aim for the healthy weight range for your height. Try to maintain your current weight, or you may need to lose weight if you are already overweight or obese. Remember to keep your weight goals within reason — you are still recovering and your weight loss or gain should be gradual. Focus on becoming active for 30–60 minutes, five to six days per week. Buy a pedometer to track how many steps you take each day. Aim for 10,000 steps (five miles) each day (2,000 steps = one mile). Studies showed that weight training is an important key to rebuilding muscle mass after cancer treatment. Women with breast cancer, in particular, required strength training to rebuild muscle mass. Interestingly, women who trained at home showed no improvement. As you look to your new life, this may be a great time to have a registered physical or occupational therapist give you guidance and suggestions on your specific needs. Eat smaller meals and snacks to limit calories if you need to lose weight. Consider having your metabolic rate evaluated by a registered dietitian. By knowing your individual calorie needs, you will be able to form an effective and individualized eating plan to reach your weight goals.

As you begin making better choices in your eating, remember that most oncology practices offer the services of a registered dietitian to help you reach your goals for healthier living. They can offer further education, support, and guidance on the benefits of nutrition for the cancer survivor.

# Q: Once I feel fine, can I return to work?

A: Following your cancer treatment, you might be looking to return to work for increased financial stability. You probably had to put your previous job on hold, or you might be planning to start a new job. Getting yourself back into the workforce often presents an opportunity to enhance your self-esteem and self-worth. For many cancer survivors, returning to work can be exciting but also present challenges. It's important not to rush into work if you're still dealing with post-treatment effects such as fatigue. You may want to consider going back to work part-time in order to pace yourself. Here are some other suggestions to consider when thinking about a return to work:

- Consult with your oncologist and get a status report on your health and any physical limitations that might present obstacles to working. Request that your doctor provide you with a statement or letter that confirms you are in good health and disease free when you are ready to return to work.

- Give careful consideration to your skills and abilities before returning to the workforce. Dealing with cancer and going through treatment can be very stressful and draining on your body. Speak with your physician once again about any job prospects that would add undue stress upon you.

- If it is a new job you are looking for, avoid compiling your resume into chronological order; this way you won't have to explain gaps in your work history. Emphasize your skills and qualifications for the job. During an interview, if you are asked, it's always best to be honest about your medical history. Respond with positive statements about your health and keep the focus on your abilities instead.

- Think about how much you want to share with your coworkers about your experience. Attitudes may vary, but it's important that you feel comfortable and at ease when talking about your cancer. Seek out other coworkers who have also dealt with cancer in the past. You may also want to consider starting a support group for cancer survivors in your company if one doesn't already exist.

- Familiarize yourself with the Americans with Disabilities Act (ADA). This law was enacted in 1992. For private and public employers with greater than 15 employees, it bans discrimination against those who have a disability, including people with cancer. Among your protections under the ADA, your employer must allow for reasonable accommodations. This means your employer must take into consideration any special needs you have on the job and make arrangements for these needs. The employer is required to modify your work schedule or provide you with the equipment necessary to perform the job. During the hiring process, employers cannot ask questions about the existence of a disability, but can inquire about your ability to perform job functions. However, the ADA also allows for certain protections for the employer, including that any arrangements that are made for the employee cannot lead to unnecessary hardship or difficulties that may cost production on the job.

## Conclusion

The first step toward moving on with your life after cancer is to realize and accept that cancer has impacted you emotionally and that you are not alone. Realize that everyone lives their life differently—therefore, there is no "normal." Recognize that cancer is now a part of your life; however, it is not your entire life. Working toward identifying the emotional impact cancer has had on your identity, your family, and your professional life is one of the first steps toward acceptance and healing. You may even find through this self-exploration that you are more in touch with your life goals and able to make the most of your life. You may have gained a unique perspective that others may not recognize.

# Glossary

**Abraxane:** See Nab-paclitaxel.

**Acquired mutations:** genetic alterations resulting from chronic physical, chemical, radiological, and natural injury to DNA; responsible for 90% of adult malignancies.

**Adenocarcinoma:** a form of cancer that develops from a malignant transformation of the cells lining a glandular organ such as the breast; almost all breast cancers are adenocarcinomas.

**Adenocarcinoma of the breast:** See above.

**Adjuvant therapy:** an additional treatment used to increase the effectiveness of the primary therapy; chemotherapy is often used as an adjuvant treatment after a mastectomy.

**Adriamycin:** the most commonly used anthracycline antibiotic-type chemotherapy.

**Alternative therapies:** unconventional cancer therapies offered as replacement to standard modalities of chemotherapy and radiation; not recognized by medical establishment or insurers, often untested but supported by personal anecdote.

**Amino acids:** specific types of chemical compounds that are the building blocks of proteins.

**Aneuploid:** having an abnormal number of sets of chromosomes; for example, tetraploid means having two paired sets of chromosomes, which is twice as many as normal; aneuploid cancer cells tend not to respond as well to therapy; aneuploidy refers to the state of being aneuploid; see also diploid and ploidy.

**Angiogenesis:** the growth of new blood vessels, a characteristic of tumors; angiogenesis is a normal biologic process that occurs in both healthy and diseased states; "angiogenesis factor" or "tumor angiogenesis factor" refers to a substance that tumors produce in order to grow new blood vessels.

**Anthracyclines:** (or anthracycline antibiotics) class of chemotherapy drugs related to antibiotics; the most common brand names include Adriamycin, Epirubicin, and Doxil.

**Aromatase:** an enzyme that converts an adrenal chemical to estrogen (estradiol or estrone); primarily found in fat cells but also found in muscle and liver cells.

**Aromatase inhibitor:** a drug that blocks an enzyme that converts an adrenal chemical to estrogen (estradiol or estrone).

**Aspiration:** the use of suction to remove fluid or tissue, usually through a fine needle (e.g., aspiration biopsy).

**Atypical ductal hyperplasia:** a precancerous overgrowth of duct cells.

**Axilla:** the anatomic name for the armpit.

**Axillary dissection:** the surgical evaluation of the axillary (armpit) by opening the axillary fascia and removing lymph nodes along the axillary vein.

**Axillary sampling:** removal of some axillary nodes without a required or formal entry of axillary fascia and dissection along the axillary vein.

**Benign:** relatively harmless; not cancerous; not malignant.

**Bilateral:** both sides; for example, a bilateral mastectomy is a mastectomy in which both breasts are removed.

**Biopsy:** sampling of tissue from a particular part of the body (e.g., the breast) in order to check for abnormalities such as cancer; removed tissue is typically examined microscopically by a pathologist in order to make a precise diagnosis of the patient's condition.

**Bisphosphonates:** class of drug used to treat bones compromised by osteoporosis or metastases.

**Bone marrow:** soft tissue in bone cavities that produces blood cells.

**Bone scan:** a technique that is more sensitive than conventional x-rays, it uses a radio labeled agent to identify abnormal or cancerous growths within or attached to bone; in the case of breast cancer, a bone scan is used to identify bone metastases; metastases appear as "hot spots" on the film; however, the absence of hot spots does not prove the absence of tiny metastases.

**BRCA:** a mutated gene associated with breast cancer. Types 1 and 2 can be routinely tested in high-risk women.

**Breast-conservation surgery:** a surgical procedure in which the cancer is removed, but the breast is spared; also called segmental mastectomy, quadrantectomy, and lumpectomy.

**Breast imaging:** techniques used to look at breast anatomy and physiology including mammogram, ultrasound, PER and MRI.

**Breast ultrasound:** a sound or sonar evaluation of the breasts useful when mammogram is not equivocal, especially in young women.

**Breast ultrasonography:** See above

**CAD (Computer Aided Detection) mammography:** A computer program that assists mammogram reading.

**Cancer:** the growth of abnormal cells in the body in an uncontrolled manner; unlike benign tumors, cancerous tumors tend to invade surrounding tissues and spread to distant sites of the body via the bloodstream and lymphatic system.

**Cancer prevention:** interventions to stop cancer before it develops.

**Cancer relapse:** the recurrence of cancer after initial treatment in a patient thought to be cancer free.

**Carcinogenesis:** the sequential genetic and molecular changes that are responsible for cellular transformations into cancer.

**Carcinoma:** a form of cancer that originates in organ tissues as a result of transformation of the epithelial cells.

**Chemoprevention:** the use of a pharmaceutical or other substance to prevent the development of cancer.

**Chemotherapy:** the use of pharmaceuticals or other chemicals to kill cancer cells; in many cases, chemotherapeutic agents kill not only cancer cells but also other cells in the body, making such agents potentially very dangerous.

**Chromosome:** a thread-like linear strand of DNA and associated proteins in the nucleus of cells; carries the genes and functions in the transmission of hereditary information.

**Clinical findings:** the combined results of exam, lab, and imaging.

**Clinical trial:** a carefully planned experiment to evaluate a treatment or a medication (often a new pharmaceutical) for an unproven use; Phase I trials are very preliminary short-term trials involving a few patients, designed to evaluate safety; Phase II trials may involve 20 to 50 patients and are designed to estimate the most active dose of a new drug and evaluate efficiency; Phase III trials involve many patients and compare a new therapy against the current standard or best available therapy to evaluate superiority.

**Collumnators:** the part of a linear accelerator that contours the radiation beam to the part of the body being treated.

**Complementary therapies:** unconventional therapies that can be effectively integrated into standard medical care but are not necessarily endorsed by the medical establishment or proven by evidence-based criteria to improve outcomes.

**Complete axillary node dissection:** the removal of all (approximately 40) axillary lymph nodes by dissecting along the axillary vein below (level 1), under (level 2), and above (level 3) the pectoralis muscle (also see axillary dissection).

**Complete response:** total disappearance of all evidence of disease; disease is no longer detected using physical examination, laboratory studies, and radiologic imaging; a criterion for evaluating the efficacy of a particular anticancer therapy (see Partial response).

**Complication:** an unexpected or unwanted effect of a treatment, pharmaceutical, or other procedure.

**Computerized axial tomography (CAT or CT scan):** a method of combining images from multiple x-rays under the control of a computer to produce cross-sectional or three-dimensional pictures of the internal organs that can be used to identify abnormalities; used for evaluating metastases of the lymph nodes or more distant soft tissue sites.

**Congenital mutations:** gene alterations that develop in utero.

**Connective tissue:** muscle, ligament, and tendon of the musculoskeletal system.

**Core biopsy:** the removal of a core of tissue from a tumor for the purpose of pathologic examination.

**CT scan:** computerized or computed tomography (see computerized axial tomography).

**Curative intent:** treatment designed with the expectation of cure.

**DCIS:** See Ductal Carcinoma in situ.

**Diagnosis:** the evaluation of signs, symptoms, and selected test results by a physician to determine the physical and biological causes of the signs and symptoms and whether a specific disease or disorder is involved.

**Differentiation:** (1) the process by which the homogenous cells of the developing embryo change into the 200+ cell types of the human being and (2) the process showing how mature (developed) the cancer cells are in a tumor; differentiated tumor cells resemble normal cells and grow at a slower rate than undifferentiated tumor cells, which lack the structure and function of normal cells and grow more aggressively.

**Diffuse metastatic:** extensive cancer spread throughout the body.

**Digital mammography:** a computer enhanced form of mammography.

**Diploid:** having one complete set of normally paired chromosomes, that is, a normal amount of DNA; a diploid number of chromosomes would equal 46, and a haploid set would equal 23 (see also ploidy, aneuploid).

**Disease-specific survival:** a clinical trial outcome that distinguishes between death from cancer vs. other causes.

**DNA:** the basic biologically active chemical that defines the physical development and growth of nearly all living organisms; a complex protein that is the carrier of genetic information.

**Docetaxel: (Taxotere):** one of the four in the taxane class of chemotherapy.

**Doxorubicin (adriamycin):** See Anthracyclines.

**Duct:** the tube-like structure of mammary tissue that transfers mothers' milk from the lobule cells to the nipple.

**Ductal carcinoma:** a nonspecific term used to describe cancer of mammary tissue.

**Ductal carcinoma in situ:** the earliest form of breast cancer before it invades through the duct wall.

**Ductal hyperplasia:** the earliest change of duct cell growth, characterized by orderly overgrowth.

**Ectoderm:** the layer of pre-embryologic cells that gives rise to skin and nerves.

**Electromagnetic spectrum:** the range of radiant energy that is distinguished by wavelength and includes therapeutic radiation, visible light, radiowaves, etc.

**Embryo:** the human in its earliest stage of intrauterine development.

**Endoderm:** the layer of cells in the developing embryo that gives rise to the body's organs.

**Enzyme:** any of a group of chemical substances that are produced by living cells and that cause particular chemical reactions to happen while not being changed themselves.

**Epithelial cell:** those cells derived from the endoderm and that comprise the organs.

**Estrogen:** a sex hormone associated with female secondary sex characteristics.

**Estrogen receptor:** the docking site on the cell for estrogen; it is a protein that can be measured and quantified.

**Excisional biopsy:** the removal of an area of diseased tissue in its entirety for submission for pathologic review.

**External beam radiation therapy:** a form of radiation therapy in which the radiation is delivered by a machine directed at the area to be radiated, as opposed to radiation given within the target tissue such as with brachytherapy.

**Faslodex: (Fulvestart):** An antiestrogen therapy.

**Fatty tissue:** tissue comprised of fat cells.

**Fine-needle aspiration:** removal of cellular material from diseased tissue via a needle for submission for pathologic review.

**FISH:** See Fluorescent in situ hybridization.

**Flow cytometry:** a measurement method that determines the fraction of cells that are diploid, tetraploid, aneuploid, etc. (ploidy status), as well as the percent of DNA undergoing synthesis (S-phase).

**Fluorescent in situ hybridization:** A laboratory technique that can identify specific DNA sequences.

**Fraction:** the portion of a fractionated radiation treatment that is delivered in a single session.

**Freedom from progression:** an outcome measurement.

**Fulvestrant:** See Faslodex.

**GAIL model:** a breast cancer incidence predictive model.

**Gamma radiation:** very short wavelength electromagnetic radiation used for therapeutic radiation.

**Gene:** a discrete DNA sequence that codes for a specific protein.

**Genetic code:** the complete gene sequence of an organism mapped out in its respective DNA code.

**Genome:** the total genetic content contained in a haploid set of chromosomes in single or multicelled organisms, in a single chromosome in bacteria, or in the DNA or RNA of viruses; an organism's genetic material.

**Genomics:** the study of genomic instability.

**Glandular:** related to organs that secrete or abosrb.

**Her-2/neu:** a gene found to be overexpressed or amplified in some breast cancer cells; evaluated routinely for both prognostic and therapeutic significance.

**HercepTest:** a rapid laboratory test for Her-2/neu activity.

**Herceptin:** the drug developed to interfere with the Her-2/neu gene/protein

**Hereditary:** inherited from one's parents and earlier generations.

**Hereditary mutations:** abnormal DNA sequences inherited from one's parents and earlier generations.

**Histologic grade:** a system that attempts to quantify a pathologist's subjective interpretation of a cell's degree of differentiation.

**Homogeneous (homogeneity):** uniform; composed of the same element; in reference to a tumor cell population, it means that the cells are of the same clone, in contrast to a mixed-cell population that would exhibit heterogeneity or be heterogeneous.

**Hormones:** biologically active chemicals that are secreted by one organ and then travel through the circulation, where they exert effort elsewhere.

**Hormone therapy:** the use of hormones, hormone analogues, and certain surgical techniques to treat disease (in this case breast cancer) either on their own or in combination with other hormones or other methods of treatment; because breast cancer may be dependent on estrogen to grow, hormonal (antiestrogen) therapy can be an effective means of alleviating symptoms and retarding the development of the disease.

**Hyperplasia:** an increase in the number of cells in an organ or tissue (see ductal hyperplasia).

**Imaging:** a radiology technique or method allowing a physician to see something that would not be visible to the unaided eye.

**Immune system:** the biological system that protects a person or animal from the effects of foreign materials such as bacteria, viruses, and other things that might make that person or animal sick.

**Implant:** (breast implant)—a type of breast reconstruction where a breast mound is recreated by the insertion of a saline filled balloon under the muscle of the chest wall.

**Incisional biopsy:** surgical removal of a piece of diseased tissue for submission for pathologic review.

**Infiltrating ductal carcinoma:** See invasive ductal carcinoma.

**Informed consent:** permission to proceed given by a patient after being fully informed of the purposes and potential consequences of a medical procedure.

**Interventional radiology:** a branch of radiology that uses imaging guidance to facilitate procedures.

**Intraductal carcinoma:** another term for DCIS.

**Invasive ductal carcinoma:** the most advanced presentation of a mammary duct cell cancer where it no longer respects the duct wall as a boundary but invades or infiltrates surrounding tissues, blood, and lymphatic channels.

**Invasive lobular carcinoma:** as above except regarding mammary lobule cells.

**Ipsilateral:** on the same side.

**Lactation:** the production of a mother's milk by mammary tissue.

**LHRH:** lutenizing hormone-release hormone.

**Ligand:** a chemical that binds to a cell surface receptor.

**Linear accelerator:** the machine that delivers external radiation.

**Lobular carcinoma in situ:** not believed to be a cancer but a defect that is associated with mammary cancer.

**Lobule:** the portion of the mammary glandular tissue that produces milk.

**Localized:** restricted to a well-defined area.

**Local recurrence:** a relapse in the conserved breast, chest wall, or axilla ipsilateral of previously treated breast cancer.

**Locally advanced:** usually refers to large tumors or those involving nodes.

**Lumpectomy:** the surgical removal of a focal area of breast cancer.

**Lupron:** an LHRH agonist useful as an antiestrogen.

**Lymph (also lymphatic fluid):** the clear fluid in which all of the cells in the body are constantly bathed; carries cells that help fight infection.

**Lymphatic system:** the tissue and organs that produce, store, and carry cells that fight infection; includes bone marrow, spleen, thymus, lymph nodes, and channels that carry lymph fluid.

**Lymphatic tissue:** See above.

**Lymphedema:** the swelling of the arm ipsilateral to the treated breast, often associated with pain and infection.

**Lymph nodes:** the small glands that occur throughout the body and that filter the clear fluid known as lymph or lymphatic fluid; lymph nodes filter out bacteria and other toxins, as well as cancer cells.

**Lymphoscintigraphy:** a radiographic imaging technique used to map lymph flow within the breast.

**Magnetic resonance:** absorption of specific frequencies of radio and microwave radiation by atoms placed in a strong magnetic field.

**Magnetic resonance imaging:** the use of magnetic resonance with atoms in body tissues to produce distinct cross-sectional and even three-dimensional images of internal organs.

**Malignancy:** a growth or tumor composed of cancerous cells.

**Malignant:** cancerous; tending to become progressively worse and to result in death; having the invasive and metastatic (spreading) properties of cancer.

**Mammary:** the glandular tissue of the breast.

**Mammogram:** an x-ray of mammary tissue.

**Mammoprint:** a multigene assay for breast cancer prognosis.

**Mamosite:** a targeted radiation delivery system for breast cancer.

**Mammotome:** a tool used to facilitate stereotactic breast biopsies.

**Margin:** normally used to mean the surgical margin, which is the outer edge of the tissue removed during surgery; if the surgical margin shows no sign of cancer, then it is a negative margin.

**Mastectomy:** surgical removal of the breast.

**Medical oncologist:** an oncologist primarily trained in the use of medicines (rather than surgery) to treat cancer.

**Menopause:** the condition associated with the decline in estrogen production during a woman's middle age.

**Mesoderm:** the middle cellular layer of the developing embryo, which gives rise to blood, muscle, and bone.

**Meta-analysis:** a statistical method that combines many related but not identical clinical trial outcomes to assess meaningful trends in patient treatment.

**Metastasis** (plural is **metastases**): a secondary tumor formed as a result of a cancer cell or cells from the primary tumor site (e.g., the breast) traveling through the blood circulation to a new site and then growing there.

**Metastasize:** spread of a malignant tumor to other parts of the body.

**Metastatic:** having the characteristics of a secondary cancer.

**Metastatic therapy:** the treatment of proven and measurable metastases.

**Microarray testing:** the study of genes and proteins likely to predict cancer risk.

**Microcalcifications:** small calcium deposits, nearly invisible without magnification, found within some areas of DCIS.

**Micrometastasis** (plural is **micrometastases**): a metastasis too small to be measured by conventional testing.

**Modified radical mastectomy:** the surgical removal of the breast and axillary lymph nodes through a single incision.

**Morbidity:** unhealthy consequences and complications resulting from treatment.

**Mutation:** a defect in a DNA nucleoside base sequence that can lead to altered gene expression.

**Nab-paclitaxel (Abraxane):** one of the Taxane class drugs approved for breast cancer treatment.

**National Surgical Adjuvant Breast and Bowel Project (NSABP):** a large clinical trial cooperative group.

**Neoadjuvant:** the use of a different kind of therapy before the use of what is considered a more definitive therapy (e.g., the use of neoadjuvant chemotherapy before surgery for breast cancer); neoadjuvant is contrasted to adjuvant, which relates to the use of another therapy after the more definitive therapy.

**Neoplasia:** the growth of cells under conditions that would tend to prevent the development of normal tissue (e.g., a cancer).

**Neoplasm:** from the Greek meaning "new growth"; an abnormal and uncoordinated growth of cells resulting in a tumor.

**Noninvasive ductal cancer:** Also called intraductal or DCIS.

**NSABP:** See National Surgical Adjuvant Breast and Bowel Project.

**Nuclear grade:** a system that attempts to quantify a pathologist's subjective interpretation of a cell's nuclear abnormality.

**Nucleoside bases:** the four characters representing the chemical code for DNA.

**Nucleus:** the dense core of the cell containing DNA.

**Oligometastatic:** isolated cancer outside the organ of origin.

**Oncologist:** a physician who specializes in the treatment of various types of cancer.

**Oncology:** the branch of medical science dealing with tumors.

**Oncotype DX:** a multigene assay for breast cancer prognosis.

**Oopherectomy:** surgical removal of ovary.

**Organ:** a group of tissues that work in concert to carry out a specific set of functions (e.g., the heart, lungs, or breast).

**Osteoporosis:** a condition characterized by the decreased density of bone.

**Overall survival:** an outcome measure of cancer treatment effectiveness.

**Paclitaxel (Taxol):** A taxane class drug.

**Palliative:** designed to relieve a particular problem without necessarily solving it; for example, palliative therapy is given in order to relieve symptoms and improve quality of life but does not cure the patient.

**Palpable:** capable of being felt during a physical examination by an experienced physician; in the case of breast cancer, this normally refers to some form of abnormality of the breast that can be felt during an examination.

**Partial breast irradiation:** technique to limit radiation exposure.

**Partial mastectomy:** See lumpectomy.

**Partial response:** a 50% or greater decline in parameters that are being used to measure anticancer activity; parameters include abnormalities found using physical exams and laboratory and radiologic studies (see Complete response).

**Pathologist:** a physician who specializes in the examination of tissues and blood samples to help decide what diseases are present and therefore how they should be treated.

**Perimenopausal:** the years of estrogen production decline that precede menopause.

**Phase I Clinical Trial:** an evaluation of a novel treatment's toxicity.

**Phase II Clinical Trial:** an evaluation of a novel treatment's efficacy.

**Phase III Clinical Trial:** an evaluation of a novel treatment's superiority.

**Placebo:** a form of safe but nonactive treatment frequently used as a basis for comparison with pharmaceuticals in research studies.

**Plasma:** the viscous fluid of blood in which the blood cells are suspended.

**Platelet:** a blood cell involved in blood clotting.

**Ploidy:** a term used to describe the number or sets of chromosomes in a cell (see Diploid and Aneuploid).

**Positron emission tomography:** a scan using a radioactive isotope that is taken up by tumor tissue, showing that the tumor is functional.

**Primary systemic:** See neoadjuvant.

**Progesterone:** a specific steroid hormone in the family of progestins secreted by the corpus luteum of the ovary and by the placenta; it acts to prepare the uterus for implantation of the fertilized ovum, to maintain pregnancy, and to promote development of the mammary glands; many tumor cells contain progesterone receptors; used in the treatment of hot flashes; an example of a progestin is Megace.

**Prognosis:** the patient's potential clinical outlook based on the status and probable course of disease; chance of recovery.

**Prognostic criteria:** features of a cancer that fall outside traditional staging criteria but nonetheless are predictive of outcome.

**Progression:** continuing growth or regrowth of the cancer.

**Prophylactic:** preventative.

**Protein:** one of three major chemical classes found in living matter along with fats and carbohydrates. The machines of cells.

**Proteinomics:** the study of proteins resulting from genomic instability.

**Protocol:** a precise set of methods by which a research study is to be carried out.

**PSA (prostate specific antigen):** a chemical found in the normal prostate gland that may elevate in the blood when the gland undergoes cancer transformation.

**Quality of life:** an evaluation of health status relative to the patient's age, expectations, and physical and mental capabilities.

**Radiant energy:** See electromagnetic spectrum.

**Radiation oncologist:** a physician who has received special training regarding the treatment of cancers with different types of radiation.

**Radiation therapy:** the use of X-rays and other forms of radiation to destroy malignant cells and tissue.

**Radical mastectomy:** the surgical removal of the breast and axillary contents as well as the pectoralis and vasculature.

**Radiotherapy:** See radiation therapy.

**Raloxifene (Evista):** a serm class antiestrogen.

**Randomized:** a feature of clinical trials whereby participants are assigned to different treatments to remove investigator bias.

**Receptor:** a docking site that interacts with a ligand (e.g., estrogen); receptors may be on the cell membrane or within the cell cytoplasm or nucleus; estrogen receptors are examples; all cells have multiple receptors.

**Reconstructive surgery:** a surgical subspecialty.

**Recurrence:** the reappearance of disease; this can be manifested clinically as findings on the physical examination or as a laboratory recurrence or as an imaging finding.

**Red blood cell:** one of three blood cell classes along with white blood cells and platelets; responsible for oxygen transport throughout the body.

**Re-excision:** the removal of suspected residual microscopic contamination after a lumpectomy.

**Regression:** the real or apparent disappearance of some or all of the signs and symptoms of cancer; the period (temporary or permanent) during which a disease remains under control, without progressing; even complete remission does not necessarily indicate cure.

**Relapse:** See cancer relapse.

**Relapse-free progression:** an outcome measure of cancer therapy.

**Remission:** the measurable repression or shrinkage of a cancer—may be qualified as partial, complete, clinical, etc.

**Resection:** surgical removal.

**Response:** a decrease in disease that occurs because of treatment; divided into complete response (remission), partial response (remission), clinical response (by exam), radiologic response (by imaging), pathologic response (by microscopic review), etc.

**Ribosome:** the organelle within a cell's cytoplasm responsible for protein synthesis.

**Risk:** the chance or probability that a particular event will or will not happen.

**RNA:** ribonucleic acid.

**Salvage:** a procedure intended to "rescue" a patient after the failure of a prior treatment; for example, a salvage mastectomy would be the surgical removal of the breast after the failure of prior radiation therapy and lumpectomy to prevent a local reoccurrence.

**Screening:** evaluating populations of people in order to diagnose disease early.

**Segmental mastectomy:** see lumpectomy.

**Selective estrogen receptor modulator (SERM):** a drug that selectively blocks one estrogen receptor but allows other receptors at specific sites to function normally with estrogen; Tamoxifen and Raloxifene are examples of SERMs—they block the estrogen receptors in the breast and uterine tissue but allow the estrogen receptor in bone tissue to be operative.

**Sensitivity:** the probability that a diagnostic test can correctly identify the presence of a particular disease assuming the proper conduct of the test; specifically, the number of true positive results divided by the sum of the true positive results and the false negative results (see specificity).

**Sentinel lymph node:** that node that is first in line to receive lymph drainage from a particular anatomic location.

**Sentinel node biopsy:** the surgical removal of the sentinel node following its identification by lymphoscintigraphy or enhancement by injected visible dye.

**SERM:** See Selective estrogen receptor modulator.

**Side effect:** a reaction to medication or treatment (most commonly used to mean an unnecessary or undesirable effect).

**Simple mastectomy:** surgical removal of the breast without disruption of the axillary fascia or underlying muscles of the chest wall.

**Specificity:** the probability that a diagnostic test can correctly identify the absence of a particular disease, assuming the proper conduct of the test; specifically, the number of true negative results divided by the sum of the true negative results and the false positive results; a method that detects 95% of true cancer cases is highly sensitive, but if it also falsely indicates that 40% of those who do not have cancer do have cancer, then its specificity is 60% (rather poor).

**S-phase:** see flow cytometry.

**Squamous cell carcinoma:** squamous epithelial cells that have undergone cancerous transformation.

**Stage:** a term used to define the size and physical extent of a cancer.

**Staging:** the process of determining extent of disease in a specific patient in light of all available information; it is used to help determine appropriate therapy.

**Stereotactic breast biopsy:** a technique using radiographic imaging to guide the biopsy of a nonpalpable lesion.

**Support drugs:** medications that have no inherent anticancer activity but improve the tolerance and safety of standard treatment.

**Surgical:** referring to surgery.

**Survival:** an outcome measure of cancer treatment effectiveness.

**Symptom:** a feeling, sensation, or experience associated with or resulting from a physical or mental disorder and noticeable by the patient.

**Systemic:** throughout the whole body; affecting the entire body.

**Systemic therapy:** a therapy designed to be effective throughout the entire body.

**Tamoxifen:** an antiestrogen treatment of the SERM type.

**Targeted therapy:** therapies designed to target unique molecular structures.

**Taxanes:** a class of chemotherapy drugs that includes brand names Taxol (paclitaxel) and Taxotere.

**Taxol:** See Paclitaxel.

**Taxotere:** See Docetaxel.

**Therapy:** the treatment of disease or disability.

**Time to progression:** an outcome measure of cancer treatment effectiveness.

**Tissues:** An organization of cells.

**TNM staging system:** a system for quantifying the extent of malignancy by numerically "grading" the size and extent of the primary tumor, the degree of involvement of lymph nodes and the presence or absence of distant spread (metastases).

**TRAM:** a reconstructive procedure that builds a breast mound from the transabdominal rectus muscle.

**Treatment:** administration of remedies to a patient for a disease.

**Tumor:** an excessive growth of cells caused by uncontrolled and disorderly cell replacement; an abnormal tissue growth that can be either benign or malignant (see Benign and malignant).

**Tykerb (Lapatinib):** an anti-VEGF drug.

**Ultrasound:** sound waves at a particular frequency (far beyond the hearing range) whose echoes bouncing off tissue can be used to image internal organs (e.g., a baby in the womb).

**Vascular tissue:** related to blood vessels.

**VEGF (vascular endothelial growth factor):** a chemical expressed in cancer cells and a target of recent therapies.

**Wavelengths:** See Electromagnetic spectrum.

**White blood cell count:** one of three classes of blood cells along with red blood cells and platelets; responsible for immune surveillance.

# Index

## I

immediate medical evaluation  27
IMMUNE SYSTEM  41
implant  52
INFILTRATING DUCTAL CARCI-
        NOMA  16
informed consent  32, 59
infrared light  47
INTERVENTIONAL RADIOLOGY  99
intraductal cancer  15
invasive cancer  21, 37, 39
INVASIVE DUCTAL CARCINOMA
        16
INVASIVE LOBULAR CANCER  16
invasive state  24
ipsilateral  43

## L

laboratory data  59
LACTATION  11
LHRH  69
LIGAND  68
LINEAR ACCELERATOR  47
LOBULAR CARCINOMA IN SITU
        16
LOBULES  11
localized breast cancer  98
LOCALLY ADVANCED  98
locoregional therapy  48, 83
Lumpectomy  4, 35, 44
LYMPHATIC SYSTEM  10, 40
lymph channels  41
lymphedema  43
lymph node  40, 58
        sampling  49
        windows to circulatory system  42
lymphoscintigraphy  44

## M

MAGNETIC RESONANCE IMAG-
        ING  27, 30
mammary cells  26
mammary tissue  11
        organization  11
        stresses  12
MAMMOGRAM  11, 15

abnormalities  26
mammography  24, 25
        CAD and digital  28
MAMMO PRINT  84
mammotome  35
MAMOSITE  48
margin  37, 49
mastectomy  4, 52
        bilateral  4
        modified radical  44
        partial  44
        radical  43, 45
            complications from  43
        segmental  44
        simple  44, 50, 53
Medical oncologists  2, 6
MENOPAUSE  12
menstrual period  12
MESODERM  8
meta-analysis  79
metastases  22, 23, 25
METASTASIS  22
metastasizes  25
metastatic  60
METASTATIC THERAPY  23, 60
Methotrexate  75
microarray testing  34
microbes  41
microcalcifications  15
MICROMETASTASES  42
micrometastasis  60
microwaves  47
milk production  11
systemic therapy  65
morbidity  84
MRI  30
musculoskeletal framework  9
mutated duct cells  16
MUTATION  14, 19

## N

NAB-PACLITAXEL  75
National Cancer Institute  82
National Comprehensive Cancer Center
        Network  82
National Surgical Adjuvant Breast and
        Bowel Project  75, 82

**Photo Credits for Background Images:**

DNA Model © Photodisc/Getty Images shown on pages 29, 58, 64, 96, 101, and 127.

Red Blood Cells © Chad Baker/Photodisc/Getty Images shown on pages 66, 41, 125, and 131.

Ripples in Calm Water © Photos.com shown on pages 92, 120, and 132.

Woman Giving a Self Breast Exam © LiquidLibrary shown on pages 24, 40, 98, and 11

Assortment of Pills (#2) © Photos.com shown on pages 74, 85, 95, 122, and 128.

The Chapter Openers are composed of all of the images listed above.